Contents

Introduction

This book of guide-lines and assignments is intended to provide material for hairdressing and beauty students following the City and Guilds Communication courses and YTS courses, and those taking the English Speaking Board Assessments in Oral Skills. I have included oral assignments since I feel it is so very important for hairdressers and beauticians to be able to communicate confidently, successfully and effectively in their area of work, and I hope these assignments will be useful. All the assignments are extremely practical and I have tried to make them as realistic as possible. My own students are allocated, on average, one and a quarter hours per week for communications; some of these assignments can be covered in one lecture period, but others will take longer to complete.

Shelagh Snell

Communications in the Salon

Practical guide-lines and assignments
for hairdressing and beauty students

SHELAGH SNELL
Lecturer in Communications
Worcester Technical College

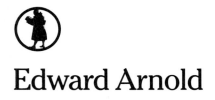

Edward Arnold

© *Shelagh Snell 1987*

First published in Great Britain in 1987 by
Edward Arnold (Publishers) Ltd, 41 Bedford
Square, London WC1B 3DQ

Edward Arnold (Australia) Pty Ltd, 80 Waverley
Road, Caulfield East, Victoria 3145, Australia

British Library Cataloguing in Publication Data

Snell, Shelagh
  Communications in the salon : practical
  guide-lines and assignments for hairdressing
  and beauty students.
  1. Communication in beauty shops
  2. Communication in hairdressing
  I. Title
  302.2   TT958

ISBN 0-7131-7512-5

Text set in 10/12 pt Century Compugraphic
by Mathematical Composition Setters Ltd,
Salisbury, Wiltshire
Printed and bound in Great Britain by
The Bath Press, Avon

Acknowledgements

I am grateful to my colleagues at Worcester Technical College for their help and encouragement in writing this book, and in particular Maire Hewitt, Janet Green, Anne Wall and other members of the hairdressing department for whose students it was originally written. My thanks are due also to Mike Wilson and David Byram-Wigfield of the Department of General Studies and Art, who have 'tried out' the assignments on their students, to Joyce Asbury of Dudley College of Technology, and to Hettie Jones, the librarian at Worcester Technical College, for their considerable support.

I am also extremely grateful to Christabel Burniston MBE for her wisdom and advice on the oral section of the book, and to Douglas Dale, chartered accountant, and James Snell, chartered architect, for their help on the assignment 'Setting up on your own'.

Finally, my thanks to Gill Owen, who has typed my work with such efficiency and good humour.

The publishers would like to thank the following for their permission to include copyright material:

Able, Humphreys Associates and Ordnance Survey for part of Worcester Street Map (p. 70); Conde Nast Publications Ltd and Penguin Books Ltd for an extract from *The Vogue Body and Beauty Book* (p. 33); Consumers Association for 'The Viewers' View' from *Which?* November 1983 (p. 2); The Econasign Co. Ltd for their stencil illustration (p. 29); Guardian Royal Exchange for their claim form (p. 7); *Health and Beauty Salon* for an extract from 'Careers in Beauty Therapy' (pp. 24–5); Letraset UK Limited for an illustration from their catalogue (p. 30); London Regional Transport for an underground map (p. 18); Office of Fair Trading for an extract from *Launderers and Dry Cleaners* (p. 11); Paris Travel Service Ltd for part of their brochure (p. 64); Rotring for an illustration from their catalogue (p. 30) and TrainLines of Britain for the London to Hereford timetable (p. 17).

Foreword

It is a great pleasure to meet, at last, a book which recognises the human and personal attributes needed at all levels in the hairdressing and beauty industry.

The efficiency and harmonious running of any such establishments depend on clear, concise and courteous communication, be it in the manager's office, at the reception desk or in the salon. The *quality* of the ever expanding hairdressing and beauty industry is shown in its personal service, however much new technology replaces human hands. In this book, Shelagh Snell sets out to help young men and women who are training for a variety of jobs within the industry, and from her wide experience as a communications lecturer in Further Education she deals with the many aspects of written and oral communication which determine effective interaction.

At the request of several Colleges of F.E. the English Speaking Board have provided a welcome addition to their existing oral assessments in the form of a syllabus specifically related to hairdressers and beauty training. Shelagh Snell's book sets out essential guidelines which will help students in their preparation for these assessments, but far beyond that, it provides valuable advice and practice for all aspirants as they meet real-life situations in an infinitely varied and demanding profession.

Christabel Burniston
President of the English Speaking Board

Assignment 1: The TV survey

After a long tiring day in the salon, a hairdresser is usually only too thankful to sink into a comfortable armchair and switch on the television set for his or her favourite programme. Sometimes, however, the set is switched on regardless of the programme, since we have the reputation of being 'A Nation of Box Watchers'.

Task 1

Read the extract on the following page, and study the data from a *Which* report.

Now answer the following questions.

1 What percentage of householders had a TV licence at the time of the Queen's Coronation?
2 This article was written in 1983. In what year was the Queen's Coronation?
3 What percentage of households had a TV licence when the wedding of Prince Charles and Lady Diana took place?
4 How many hours of TV programmes are broadcast each day?
5 What is the average length of viewing time per day in the UK?
6 How many hours per day, on average, does a Norwegian spend watching TV?
7 How many countries spend, on average, more than 3 hours per day watching TV?
8 How many countries spend, on average, 2 hours per day or less watching TV?

9 What percentage of people were more satisfied with BBC 1 programmes in 1983 than in 1981?
10 (a) What percentage of people were very dissatisfied with BBC 2 programmes in 1983?
   (b) Is this greater or less than in 1981?
11 What increase of people who were fairly satisfied with ITV programmes is shown in 1983 compared with 1981?
12 Does the Channel 4 figure show that people generally are satisfied with or are dissatisfied by the programmes shown on that Channel?

Task 2

Design a questionnaire for random distribution in order to test opinion on TV programmes today. You should aim to find out
(a) popularity of particular programmes,
(b) hours spent watching TV
(c) differences in popularity between channels,
(d) what people want from TV,
(e) whether TV generally is less popular today than in 1983.

Task 3

Your findings should be presented in the form of a short report.

THE VIEWERS' VIEW
WHAT WE THINK OF OUR TV PROGRAMMES

Just 30 years ago, the Queen's Coronation was televised by our single, black-and-white TV channel and watched by about 21 million people. Around 15 per cent of households had a TV licence, and the only available channel was broadcasting a total of about five hours of programmes a day. Video recorders were science fiction.

In 1981, about 40 million people in Britain watched the wedding of Charles and Diana, broadcast simultaneously and in colour on three television channels. Around 95 per cent of households had a TV licence. We now have four colour channels which broadcast a total of about 50 hours of programmes a

day. The vast majority of us watch television seven days a week; on average, we watch between three and four hours a day. Nearly one in five households has a video recorder. Watching TV has become our most time-consuming leisure activity.

This report turns the spotlight on the sort of service you think you're getting. What do you think of the programmes you receive? Are you getting value for money? What do you want to see more or less of on your screens? Has the service got better or worse over the last two years? And how do you complain if you think you're getting a raw deal?

What we did for this report
This report is based on two surveys we carried out among the general public. The first was undertaken in the spring of 1981 when nearly 2,000 out of 4,000 randomly selected people returned a long questionnaire which we sent them about their TV viewing; the second, undertaken earlier this year, asked the same questions of the same people to see how attitudes and viewing behaviour had changed. Over 1,300 replied, and some of the results were surprising. We checked and confirmed that the 1981 replies of these 1,300 were no different from the replies of the 2,000 as a whole.

A NATION OF BOX WATCHERS

According to one report earlier this year, the British watch more television each day than any other Western European country (see the Diagram). But, as many informed and sometimes worried reports from the broadcasting bodies have told us, our viewing is declining. This is certainly confirmed in our own research: the average daily viewing time among our sample is now about three hours a day. Two years ago, it was about 3 hours 40 minutes — which means that, on average the British TV viewer is watching five hours less television a week. Why?

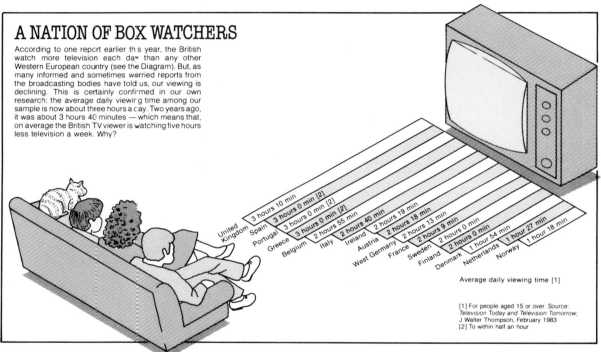

United Kingdom	3 hours 10 min
Spain	3 hours 0 min [2]
Portugal	3 hours 0 min [2]
Greece	3 hours 0 min [2]
Belgium	2 hours 55 min
Italy	2 hours 40 min
Ireland	2 hours 19 min
Austria	2 hours 18 min
West Germany	2 hours 13 min
France	2 hours 9 min
Sweden	2 hours 0 min
Finland	2 hours 0 min
Denmark	1 hour 54 min
Netherlands	1 hour 27 min
Norway	1 hour 18 min

Average daily viewing time [1]

[1] For people aged 15 or over. Source: *Television Today and Television Tomorrow*; J Walter Thompson, February 1983
[2] To within half an hour

HOW YOU RATE THE CHANNELS

Why are you watching less TV? One possibility is that you are voting with your feet because you think that the standard of programmes on offer is falling. The Chart below shows how satisfied you are with each channel now compared with two years ago. You can see that, far from falling, the satisfaction ratings have improved

appreciably 14% are *more* satisfied with BBC1 programmes than two years ago, 6% with BBC2, 10% with ITV.

You can see also that, overall, you are less satisfied with the output from ITV and, in particular, Channel 4 than with BBC output. This preference is confirmed by

the answers to our questions on your overall favourite channel — BBC1 is the winner (preferred by 47%), with ITV second (40%), while BBC2 (11%) and Channel 4 (2%) trail well behind.

Satisfaction with the programmes offered

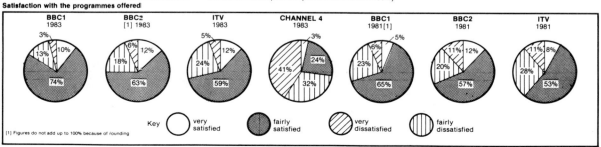

BBC1 1983	BBC2 [1] 1983	ITV 1983	CHANNEL 4 1983	BBC1 1981[1]	BBC2 1981	ITV 1981
3% / 13% / 10% / 74%	6% / 18% / 12% / 63%	5% / 24% / 12% / 59%	3% / 41% / 24% / 32%	5% / 6% / 23% / 65%	11% / 20% / 12% / 57%	11% / 28% / 8% / 53%

Key: ○ very satisfied | ● fairly satisfied | ▨ very dissatisfied | ▥ fairly dissatisfied

[1] Figures do not add up to 100% because of rounding

Guide-lines on the business letter

Basic rules

1 *Style*

(a) Aim for sincerity and friendliness, but not familiarity.
(b) Keep to the point, but avoid being curt.
(c) Always be courteous, never 'off-hand'. Even when you 'reprimand' someone by letter, e.g. in a letter of complaint, there is never any excuse for rudeness.
(d) Make quite sure that all your facts are correct. Be efficient.
(e) Always use clear, simple and straight-forward language. Avoid jargon and words you think sound impressive; they usually sound rather pompous.
(f) If you are replying to a letter — always start by thanking the sender, e.g.

Dear Mr. Jones,

Thank you for your letter dated June 5th . . .

2 *Layout*

(a) The appearance of your letter is very important indeed. The layout should always be well balanced and pleasing to look at.
(b) Consider the size of the paper you're using, and 'lay' the words on it carefully, avoiding a squashed or crowded look. Make sure there is a margin all round the letter, and that there are no great gaps left at the top or bottom of the paper.
(c) Take note of the personal preferences of the person for whom you are writing. Does he, or she, like letters to be *fully blocked*, i.e. all the typed entries (apart from his, or her, address) to begin from the left hand margin, with no indenting of paragraphs, or *semi-blocked*, with the paragraphs indented and the closing of the letter centrally placed?

3 *Punctuation*

It has become common practice to type business letters nowadays with the minimum of punctuation. Commas and full stops are used to make the sentences 'make sense', but other old established marks of punctuation such as the apostrophe are fast disappearing. It should be noted, however, that a great many people regard this not as time-saving (which is the intention) but as a sign of sloppiness, and a further example of the degeneration of our language; so take note of the personal preferences of the person for whom you are writing the letter, and if he or she likes letters to be traditionally punctuated, look carefully at the example on the following page.

The traditional method of punctuating a letter

4 *Greetings and endings*

(a) If you know the name of the person to whom you are writing, it is discourteous not to use it in the greeting, unless the name constitutes the name of a firm or company in which case you would use 'Dear Sir', 'Sirs', or 'Dear Madam'.

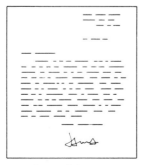

A good layout

3

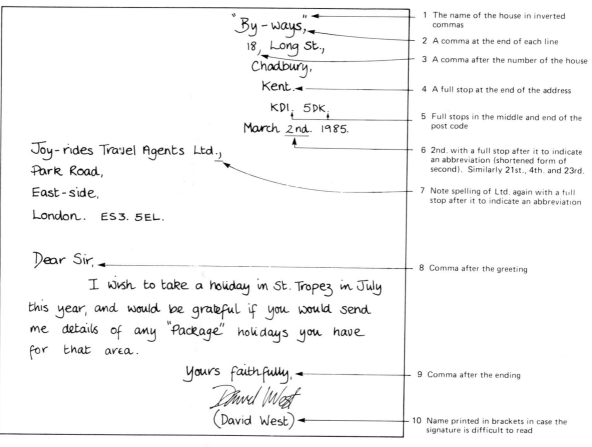

Letter diagram with annotations:

Address (top right):
"By-ways",
18, Long St.,
Chadbury,
Kent.
KD1. 5DK.
March 2nd. 1985.

Recipient (left):
Joy-rides Travel Agents Ltd.,
Park Road,
East-side,
London. ES3. 5EL.

Dear Sir,

    I wish to take a holiday in St. Tropez in July this year, and would be grateful if you would send me details of any "Package" holidays you have for that area.

Yours faithfully,
David West
(David West)

Annotations:
1 The name of the house in inverted commas
2 A comma at the end of each line
3 A comma after the number of the house
4 A full stop at the end of the address
5 Full stops in the middle and end of the post code
6 2nd. with a full stop after it to indicate an abbreviation (shortened form of second). Similarly 21st., 4th. and 23rd.
7 Note spelling of Ltd. again with a full stop after it to indicate an abbreviation
8 Comma after the greeting
9 Comma after the ending
10 Name printed in brackets in case the signature is difficult to read

(b) Use the ending 'Yours sincerely' on the following occasions:
  (i) If you have met the person to whom you are writing;
  (ii) If you have had previous correspondence with them;
  (iii) If you have been instructed to write to a specific person.

(c) The ending 'Yours faithfully' always goes with: Dear Sir, Sirs, Madam, Mesdames.

Some examples

(a) You are answering an advertisement for a job and have been instructed to write for further details to:
    Jane Archdale,
    'Hair Design',
    Wigfield Street,
    London. W 1.
You have never met Jane Archdale before, but you have been asked to write to her specifically so your letter will begin: *Dear Ms. Archdale*, and end: *Yours sincerely,*.

(b) You are writing to your previous headmaster (James Black) for a reference. Quite clearly you know the person to whom you are writing so you start your letter:
Dear Mr. Black, and end it: *Yours sincerely,*.

(c) You are writing to:
    Beauty Parlour Products Ltd.,
    5, Oakley Road,
    Lowfields,
    Berks.
to order some equipment for your salon. Beauty Parlour Products Ltd., is the name of a firm or company so you will write: *Dear Sirs,* and end your letter: *Yours faithfully,*.

Notes

1 The second letter of any correspondence usually carries the ending *Yours sincerely,* since the 'ice has been broken' and you are now deemed to know (slightly) the person to whom you are writing.

2 *Yours* always starts with a capital *Y,* followed by a small *f* and *s* for *faithfully* and *sincerely*.

Assignment 2: The missing ear-ring

You help to manage a hairdressing salon in a seaside resort where many of your customers are holiday-makers. One day you receive a telephone call from a Mrs. Haslam who claims to have lost a valuable sapphire ear-ring, presumably by theft, when having her hair shampooed and set in your salon. One of your assistants remembers seeing the ear-rings at the side of the wash-basin so it seems probable that Mrs. Haslam's story is correct.

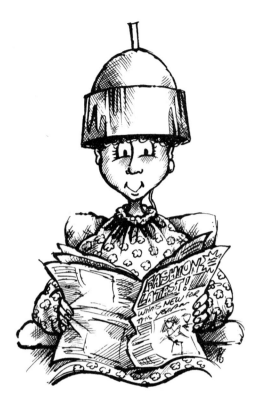

Task 1

Either by writing, or by direct approach, see if you can obtain a Theft Claim Form from an insurance company, and complete it. (Otherwise, use the one illustrated as a guide and design your own.)

Before you post the form to the insurance company, you and your staff decide to have a last search of the salon, and you find the missing ear-ring down the side of the chair Mrs. Haslam sat in when she was under the drier.

Task 2

Write an appropriate letter to Mrs. Haslam to accompany the missing ear-ring which you are returning.

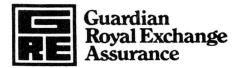

CLAIM FORM FOR FIRE THEFT MONEY AND ALL RISKS POLICIES

Policy No._____ | Branch or Agent to whom
you paid your last premium_____

Name of Insured_____

Address (Private) _____   Tel. No. { Home _____

_____   { Business_____

_____   Postcode _____

Address (Business)_____   Postcode _____

Trade or Occupation (if more than one state all) _____

Situation of premises or place where loss or damage occurred _____

Date of loss or damage_____ Time_____ a.m./p.m.

Explain fully how the loss or damage occurred_____

_____

_____

_____

_____

_____

_____

_____

_____

_____

_____

_____

_____

_____

ADDITIONAL QUESTIONS FOR THEFT MONEY AND ALL RISKS CLAIMS.

When was the loss or damage discovered?   Date_____ Time_____a.m./p.m.

By whom was the discovery made?_____

When was the property last seen?   Date_____ Time_____a.m./p.m.

By whom was it last seen?_____

When were the police notified?_____ Address of Police Station_____

Have any other steps been taken to recover the property?_____

PLEASE ANSWER THE FOLLOWING QUESTIONS IF THE CLAIM IS IN RESPECT OF A THEFT AT YOUR

OWN PREMISES

Total value of contents of premises at time of theft £_____ Are the premises, or any part, let or sub-let?_____

How many nights have the premises been unoccupied during the past year?_____

Was anyone in the premises at the time of the theft?_____ If so, please give names and addresses_____

_____

_____

What steps have you or are you taking to prevent a recurrence?_____

_____

ZC33 (7 83)   (P T O)

Assignment 3: The very awkward customer

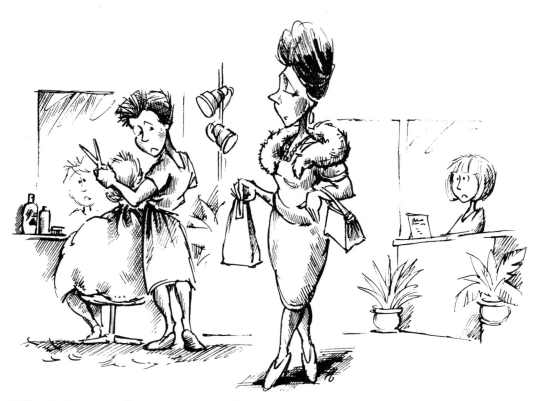

Mrs Gillespie is a regular customer at Martyne's Salon, and everyone groans when they see her coming. The trouble is that Mrs. Gillespie, many years ago, trained as a hairdresser herself, and thinks she knows better than anyone else at Martyne's. She quite sincerely believes that she can cut better, shampoo better, set hair better and perm hair better than anyone else, and although she had no training in 'beauty care', she certainly thinks she knows far more than the very able and intelligent beautician who works at Martyne's Salon.

On this particular occasion, Mrs. Gillespie is having her hair shampooed by Sarah, normally rather a shy but very pleasant young assistant who has worked at Martyne's for just over a year. Today, however, she seems quieter than usual and when Mrs. Gillespie starts complaining yet again, Sarah suddenly 'snaps'.

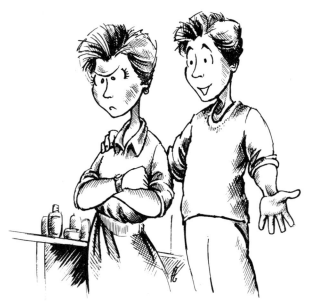

Task 1 (Group role-play)

Adopt the characters in Martyne's Salon —
there will be others apart from Mrs. Gillespie
and Sarah — and improvise the situation.

Task 2 (Role-play for 2 people)

Imagine you are the Manager/ess of Martyne's
Salon. You are worried about Sarah losing her
temper with Mrs. Gillespie and clearly must
talk to her . . .

Task 3 (Role-play for 2 people)

Imagine you are a close friend of Sarah. You
are also worried about her. See if you can find
out what's wrong.

9

Assignment 4: Taken to the cleaners

You have just collected a batch of hairdressing gowns from the cleaners and find that at least 3 of the gowns have been torn and that the stains on some of them are still apparent.

Task 1

Read the extract opposite from the Office of Fair Trading's pamphlet *Launderers and Dry Cleaners*, and answer the following questions:

1 If a laundry or dry cleaners displays the 'ABLC member' sign in their window, you know that
   (a) you will get a cheap service
   (b) you are protected by a code of practice
   (c) you will be compensated if the washing machine in the launderette ruins your clothes.

2 The term 'code of practice' means
   (a) standards of service
   (b) instruction for use
   (c) a system of coding known to the manufacturer

3 Members of the ABLC should
   (a) display a notice which states: 'Articles left with us are deposited solely at the owner's risk.'
   (b) pay you fair compensation if they lose any garment you have left with them.

4 The term 'fair compensation' means
   (a) the cost of a replacement article
   (b) the worth of the article at the time you gave it to them
   (c) the second-hand value of the article, plus a contribution towards the cost of a new replacement.

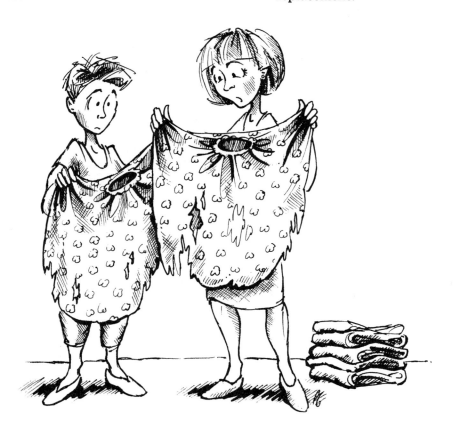

Good news from the cleaning industry

Dry cleaners and launderers are trying to make sure that whenever you use their services you get a fair deal. They have also come up with a simple procedure for dealing with your complaints.

The Code of Practice

Their professional association, the Association of British Laundry, Cleaning and Rental Services Ltd (ABLCRS), with the Office of Fair Trading, has produced a Code of Practice which lays down the standards of service its members should give you.

The main points of the Code are set out in this leaflet and cover cleaning, laundering, dyeing and repairs. *The Code does not apply to launderettes or coin-operated dry cleaners.*

Over 75 per cent of launderers and dry cleaners in England, Scotland and Wales belong to the ABLCRS and you will know your launderer or dry cleaner is a member, and that you are protected by the Code, when you see this sign.

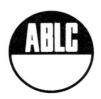

How the code will help you

Compensation

Members of the ABLCRS have agreed not to restrict their legal liability for negligence, so you should *not* see notices in shops or on the backs of tickets which say things like 'Articles left with us are deposited solely at owner's risk' or 'Compensation shall be limited to 20 times the laundry charge'.

This means that if ABLCRS members negligently lose, destroy or damage something they have accepted for processing they will pay you fair compensation. That is, what the article was worth at the time you gave it to them, allowing for loss of value due to wear but partly reflecting the cost of buying a new one. If they damage an article and it can be repaired, they will pay the cost of repair, up to the value of the item at the time.

ABLCRS members will, where the article in question is not covered by your own insurance policy, pay fair compensation for loss or damage caused by fire or burglary while it is in their care.

Occasionally a launderer or dry cleaner may feel than an item might be damaged by normal processing – in such a case you may be asked to give written acknowledgement accepting the risk of damage.

Among the possible causes of damage for which dry cleaners or launderers are not responsible are: faulty manufacture, wear and tear, and misuse by the customer.

2

5 If a fire at the cleaners or laundry destroys a garment belonging to you, they will
   (a) replace the garment
   (b) notify your insurance company
   (c) pay you fair compensation if your insurance policy does not cover the loss.
6 Launderers are not responsible for
   (a) faulty manufacture
   (b) loss through burglary
   (c) the use of incorrect cleaning fluids

Task 2

Your cleaners display the ABLC sign in their shop. How should they now deal with your hairdressing gowns?

Task 3

Imagine that you are still not satisfied with your gowns. You take the advice given in the leaflet, and write a formal letter of complaint to:
   The Manager,
   Quick-clean Services,
   25, Brewer's Lane,
   Brixham,
   Devon. DV1 4BH

Task 4

Try to obtain a copy of *Launderers and Dry Cleaners* from one of the following:
   Citizens Advice Bureau
   Consumer Advice Centre
   Trading Standards or Consumer Protection
      Department
   Public Library
   College Library
Keep it for reference: you never know, you may find it very useful one day.

Guide-lines on using the telephone

The telephone is one of the most widely used and yet one of the most feared instruments of our daily lives. Time and time again students (and indeed many adults) have said 'I hate the telephone', with a heartfelt emphasis on the word 'hate'. Why do people hate this piece of machinery so much? They hate it because it is so impersonal, because it is impossible to see the reaction of the person at the other end of the line (sometimes a distinct advantage!), and because it is impossible to make contact. The only way in which we can communicate when we use the telephone is by voice and ear. We cannot use our sight and we cannot use our hands and so our voice becomes very important indeed. It is worth noting that people who

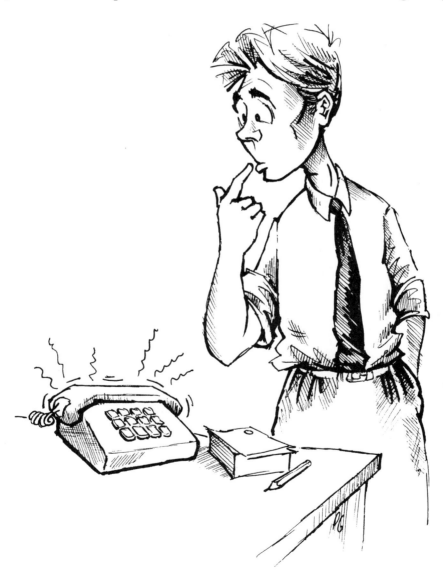

use the telephone a great deal are very seldom afraid of it. Familiarity should not breed contempt, but 'practice' in this case really does 'make perfect'.

First, remember that the telephone is the 'front' of every organisation, and the person who answers the telephone is the very first contact the caller has with that organisation. So it is very important indeed to answer the telephone correctly.

Answering the telephone

1 *The wrong way*
- *Do not* pick up the receiver, breathe heavily and wait for the caller to speak first.
- *Do not* pick up the receiver and say 'Hello!' or 'Hi' or anything casual.
- *Do not* pick up the receiver and say 'Yes?' (We have all experienced these faults at some time or other.)

2 *The right way*
- *Do* pick up the receiver and say 'Good morning', 'Good afternoon', or 'Good evening' (whichever the case may be), identify your place of work, and add 'Can I help you?'. E.g., 'Good morning. Upper Cut Hairdressing Salon, can I help you?'
- *Do* remember that it reassures the caller when you repeat the important part of the call: names, addresses, times, dates.
- *Do* try to avoid using the expression 'O.K.'. We all do it but it's a very bad habit to get into.

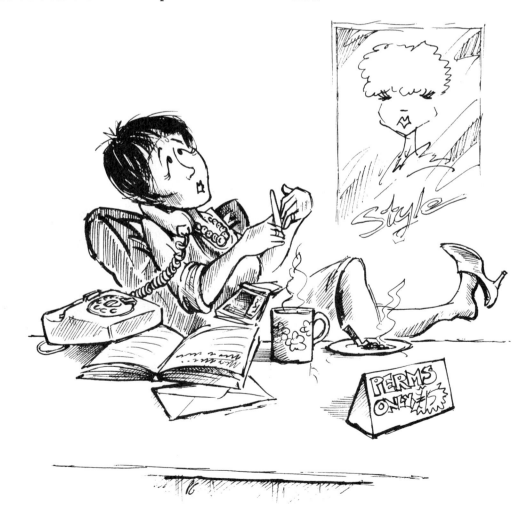

14

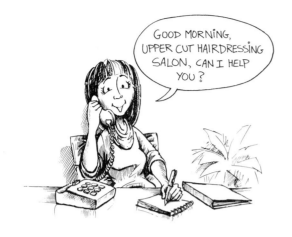

- *Do* use the caller's name when you learn it and remember to finish a call politely.
  E.g., 'Thank you for calling, Mr. Perks. We look forward to seeing you at 9 o'clock on Friday morning. Goodbye.'
Note: 'Goodbye', not 'cheerio' or 'Bye now' or anything casual.

Some situations for practice (one student to make the call, one to receive it)

1 You wish to make a hairdressing appointment for a particular date with a particular hairdresser who unfortunately is not available for the day you require. Can you reach a solution by telephone?

2 You have a rather difficult client called Mrs. Prim who rings up to say that the day after she had been to your salon for a perm, her hair had turned green! She is, perhaps understandably, rather upset. Can you deal with the situation?

3 You receive a telephone call from a young client who is very worried about the condition of her hair (it is very dry and brittle, with split ends). Can you help her?

4 You receive a telephone call from a young client who wishes to make an appointment to have her hair dyed yet again. You know this particular client, and you also know that she is ruining her hair by excessive use of peroxide. Can you tactfully dissuade her?

5 You wish to remake a hairdressing appointment. Make the appropriate telephone call.

6 You have ordered a quantity of setting lotion to replenish your stock from your wholesaler and a large quantity of neutraliser has been delivered instead, which you discover when you open the consignment some time later. Ring the wholesaler ...

7 You receive a telephone call from a client who wishes to speak to a colleague of yours, who unfortunately is not available at that particular moment. You suggest that your colleague rings the client back in an hour's time, or perhaps you could take a message for your colleague ...?

8 You wish to visit the 'Hair and Beauty Fair' in London. Ring British Rail and find out train details. Is there perhaps a 'cheapday excursion'? Will you be able to have a snack on the journey? Do you have to change trains at all?

9 Mrs. Smith rings your salon one day in a state of some agitation. She has lost her handbag and thinks she may have left it on a chair in your reception area. You have, in fact, found a handbag, but is it Mrs. Smith's?

10 You are very busy in the salon one morning just before Christmas when a colleague slips on some spilt setting lotion and it looks as though she may have broken her leg. You must ring for an ambulance ...

11 You see an advertisement in the local newspaper which states 'Part-time staff wanted for Saturdays and busy holiday periods — would suit college student. Telephone for details: Jo's Salon (0516) 591.' You decide to telephone ...

12 A representative rings you one day wanting to make an appointment to show you literature on some new solariums and to persuade you to invest in one for your salon. Are you interested? If so, make the necessary appointment. if not, can you courteously dismiss the rep?

Assignment 5: A visit to London

You are working in a hairdressing and beauty salon which has recently opened in Herefordshire. You are intending to visit London for the January sales, and the manager of your salon asks you to collect some equipment from a shop near Covent Garden for him. You decide to travel to London on the following Friday from your nearest station, Ledbury.

Task 1

Study the timetable and answer the following questions:

1 Which train would you catch in order to reach London at about 10.00 a.m.?
2 At which London station will you arrive?

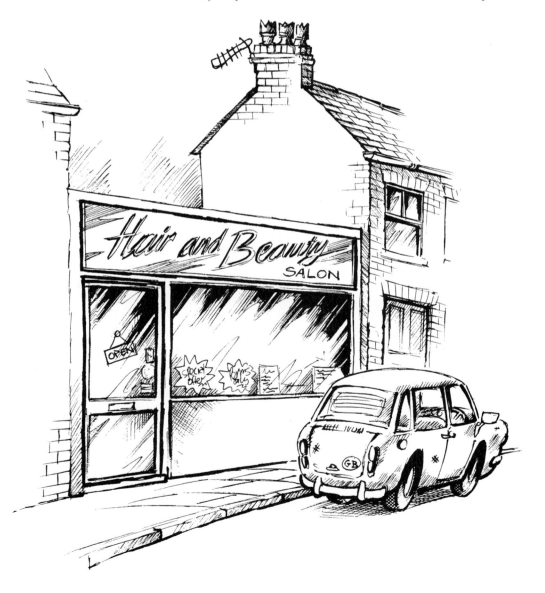

		Q	2 / B		D	P		N	N	N		H	125 N / J	N	N	H	
Hereford R	♂	03 41j	06 05	—	—	—	07 05	—	08 00	07 15	09 32	09 40x	11 46	12 25j	15 09	16 37	17 46	18 45
Ledbury	♂	—	06 21	—	—	—	07 21	—	08 21	—	09 58	—	—	12 41x 13 48x	—	16 56	17 48x	19 05
Colwall	♂	—	06 29	—	—	—	07 29	—	08 29	—	10 06x	—	—	12 49x 13 56x	—	17 04	17 53x	19 13
Great Malvern	♂	—	06 34	—	—	—	07 34	—	08 34	—	10 12x	—	—	13 43 15 30x	—	17 16	17 56x	19 22
Malvern Link	♂	—	06 38	—	—	—	07 38	—	08 38	—	10 15x	—	—	13 46 15 33x	—	17 19	18 07x	19 33
Worcester Foregate Street	♂	—	06 49	—	—	—	07 49	08 09	08 49	—	10 55	—	13 56	15 55	—	17 31	18 16	19 38
Worcester Shrub Hill R	♂	—	06 53	07 00	—	—	07 53	—	08 53	—	11 00	—	14 00	16 04	—	17 38	—	20 15
Pershore	♂	—	—	—	—	—	—	—	09 02	—	11 09	11 10	—	16 13	—	17 47	—	19 47
Evesham	♂	—	—	07 09	—	—	07 16	08 09	09 13	—	11 20	11 20	14 16	16 23	—	17 57	—	19 57
Honeybourne	♂	—	—	07 16	—	—	—	09 20	—	11 27	11 27	—	16 30	—	—	20 20
Moreton-in-Marsh	♂	—	06 15	07 23	07 29	—	—	09 36	11 50	11 50	14 33	16 46	—	18 04	20 20
Kingham	♂	—	06 23	07 38	07 38	—	—	09 45	11 58	11 58	14 40	16 55	18 20	18 29	20 29
Charlbury	♂	—	06 37	07 48	07 48	—	08 03	09 55	12 09	12 09	14 50	17 05	18 39	18 55	20 39
Oxford S	♀	—	07 00	08 17	08 03	08 32	08 59	09 42	10 11	10 29	11 15p 11 27b	12 27	13 12	14 31w 16 07	17 57	19 13	20 19	21 03
Didcot	♀	07 17	07 21	08 48	—	08 54	—	—	10 29	11 48 13 02	13 31	14 38	15 07	17 53b 20 15	21 06	22 18
Reading E S	♀	07 30	07 40 08 33	09 08	09 08	09 37	10 15	10 58	11 53	13 29	15 07	17 53	18 05	19 55 20 15	21 33	22 17v
Paddington	♀	08 00	08 10 09 07	09 37	10 58	11 27	12 21	13 29	14 07	15 07	18 30	18 34	19 13	20 32 20 48	21 49r	23 01

Notes

A Also stops Handborough 17 40, Combe 17 43, Finstock 17 49, Ascott-under-Wychwood 18 00, Shipton 18 04

B Also stops Shipton 06 28, Ascott-under-Wychwood 06 31, Finstock 06 40, Combe 06 46, Handborough 06 49

C Also stops Shipton 07 33, Ascott-under-Wychwood 07 37, Finstock 07 47, Combe 07 52, Handborough 07 56

D Also stops Shipton 07 58, Ascott-under-Wychwood 08 02, Finstock 08 12, Combe 08 17, Handborough 08 21

E Railair links with Heathrow and Gatwick airports available to/from Reading. See separate panels for details

G Also stops Shipton 10 15, Ascott-under-Wychwood 10 18, Finstock 10 29, Combe 10 35, Handborough 10 39

H Via Swindon. Service scheduled to be operated by InterCity 125 between Paddington and Swindon and vice versa

J **Cotswold & Malvern Express**

N Via Newport. Service scheduled to be operated by InterCity 125 between Paddington and Newport

P Change at Cheltenham Spa. Service scheduled to be operated by InterCity 125 between Cheltenham and Paddington

Q Via Newport

R Seats may be reserved on certain trains from this station

S Seats may be reserved from this station through the computerised seat reservation system on certain connecting services between Paddington, Reading and Oxford, also on most services between Paddington, Reading and Swindon (note H) and between Paddington, Reading and Newport (note N), also on through trains denoted by S at the head of the column

a Arrival time

b Change at Oxford

c By changing at Oxford, passengers may depart at 15 22

d Departure time

e By changing at Oxford, passengers may depart at 16 42

f Change at Didcot

g By changing at Didcot, passengers may depart at 21 29

h Sunday mornings from 6 January arrive 00 19

j Tuesdays to Fridays dep 03 49

k By changing at Oxford, passengers may depart at 16 45

m Change at Swindon and Newport. InterCity 125 between Swindon and Newport only

n Change at Oxford and Didcot

p By changing at Oxford, passengers may arrive at 10 51

q Special 'bus connection

r Change at Oxford and Reading

s Special 'bus connection between Gloucester and Swindon and vice versa

t By changing at Reading, passengers may arrive at 21 35

v By changing at Oxford, passengers may arrive Reading 21 53, Paddington 22 27

w Change at Newport and Swindon

x Second class only

y Change at Cheltenham Spa

z Change at Bristol Parkway and Newport

§ Special 'bus connection between Worcester and Gloucester and vice versa

2 Second Class only

125 Service scheduled to be operated by InterCity 125 for all or part of journey

FO Fridays only

⊡ Drinks and cold snacks available for whole or part of journey

① Hot dishes to order, also drinks and cold snacks available, for whole or part of journey

S Seats may be reserved on this train through the computer seat reservation system. Reservations may be made at London Paddington, Reading or Oxford, or at other principal British Rail Travel Centres throughout the Western Region.

British Rail car parks are provided at all stations shown in this folder except Worcester Foregate Street.

TRANSPORT USERS CONSULTATIVE COMMITTEE
If you have a complaint about British Rail services that has not been dealt with to your satisfaction, your local Transport Users Consultative Committee, set up by Parliament, will help. The address is on the T.U.C.C. notice at railway stations and is in the telephone book.

The British Railways Board accepts no liability for any inaccuracy in these tables which may be altered or cancelled at short notice, particularly during public holiday periods.

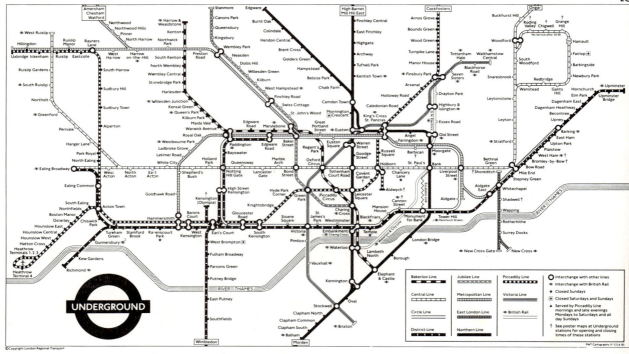

LRT U/G Map Reg. User No. 86/E/353

3 Will you be able to have a cooked breakfast on the train?

4 Your friend wants to visit a relation in Pershore the same morning. Which is the earliest train she can catch from Ledbury?

5 What does the letter 'R' mean beside the name of Hereford and Worcester Shrub Hill?

6 What is the name of the service identified by the initial 'J'?

Task 2

Your train arrives in London on time, and now you have to make your way to Covent Garden. You study the map of the London Underground and realise you cannot travel there without changing trains once. Answer the following questions:

1 How many stations will you go through before you change trains?

2 What is meant by an 'interchange station'?

3 Name the first station you should come to.

4 At which station will you change trains?

5 What will be the destination of your new train?

6 How many more stations will you come to before you reach Covent Garden?

Task 3

Write a letter to a friend in hospital telling them about your trip to London (which was very enjoyable until something went drastically wong!).

Task 4

What was the 'equipment' you had to collect? Without actually naming it, write an account of how you would use it.

Task 5

Read your account to the rest of the group. Can they guess what the piece of equipment is?

Assignment 6: The new apprentice (1)

The situation

A new apprentice is about to join your salon and your employer has assigned him/her to your care, asking you to plan an induction to the work and running of the establishment.

Task 1

Assuming that the new apprentice already knows details of pay, hours of work and holidays, make a list of all the other essential information he/she should be given.

Task 2

Describe 4 different characters the new apprentice is likely to meet during the day.

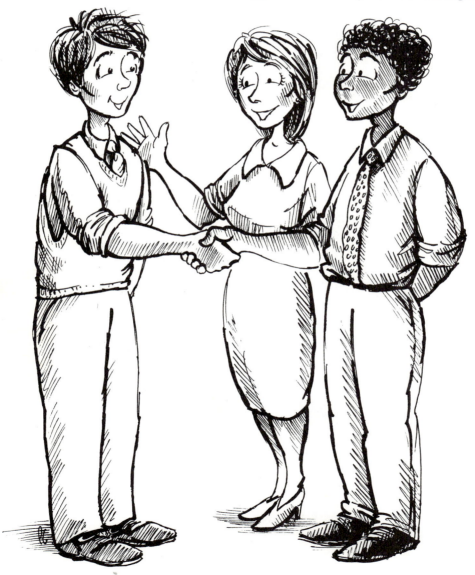

Assignment 7: The new apprentice (2)

Imagine that *you* are the new apprentice in the salon. How did you feel on your first day at work? What did you do? Whom did you meet?

Task 1

Write a letter to a friend describing your new job and your first day there.

Task 2

Write a set of instructions describing, step by step, how you would perform one of the skills you have learned.

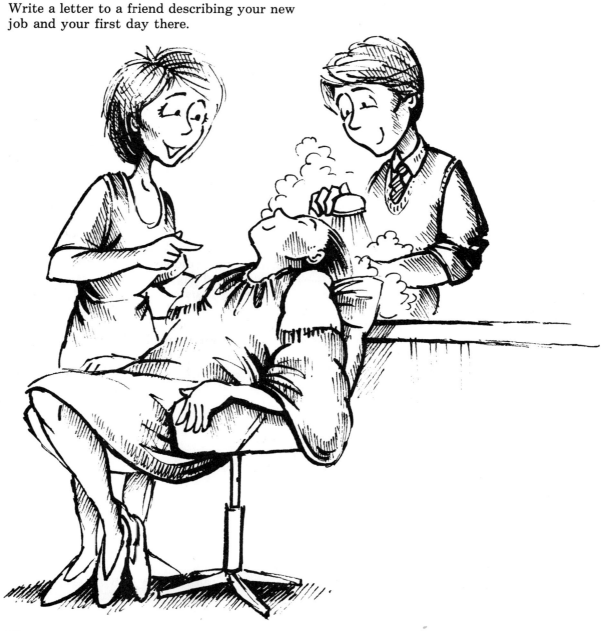

Guide-lines on applying for a job

If you look at the advertisements on the next page, some of them ask you to 'apply in writing', and some of them ask you to 'contact' someone, which could mean a telephone call, or a letter, or possibly filling in a job application form. The most important thing to remember is that your particular application will be only one of a great many, and that the badly or carelessly written, misspelt form or letter will almost certainly find its way very quickly into the wastepaper basket! So — make sure that the presentation is good, and that the spelling and grammar are correct.

The letter

This should contain the following information: age, status (married or single), names of 'secondary' schools and colleges attended (no further details needed in the letter itself — you will write these on a separate sheet of paper and attach it to the letter), details of your experience relevant to the job, and something about yourself — your interests or hobbies — which would help a future possible employer to learn something about you as a person. The whole object of writing the letter is to make a possible employer want to interview you. So — if you want to get a job — get the application right.

The form

This should be completed in pencil first to make quite sure that you haven't made any mistakes. Read intructions carefully. Where you are told to use 'block capitals' — use them! Where you are asked to fill in details of your interests or hobbies — please be careful what you write! A student of mine when filling in an application form for a job as a typist wrote that she was 'interested in all-night discos and riding pillion on her boyfriend's motor bike' — a comment hardly designed to fill a future employer with confidence!

The telephone call

The notes on 'using the telephone' apply equally here. Be confident — at this stage you have everything to gain and nothing to lose. Be polite — sometimes shyness can make people sound rude. Be positive — remember that you are ringing up to inquire about the job and then take it from there.

The C.V. (Curriculum Vitae)

This should be presented on a separate sheet of paper to be enclosed with a letter of application. It should contain full details of your schools (other than primary schools), and colleges and details of examinations taken and their results. (Only give these when you have been successful, there is no point in giving details of examinations you have failed!). You should also give full details of the contributions you have made to your school or college. For example — did you take part in any play or production of any kind? Were you a member of any games team or did you play for the school band or orchestra? Did you take a prominent part in any fund-raising activity? Do not under-present yourself! All this information should be neatly tabulated so that it can be very easily read and understood, under appropriate headings.
Now:

Task 1
Write your own C.V.

Task 2
Look at the advertisements on page 22. Choose one of them and apply for the job.

Task 3
See if you can get some job application forms (your local Job Centre may be able to help you here) and practise filling them in.

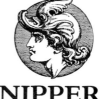

22

Guide-lines on the interview

You have applied for a job and have been selected for an interview!

This is one of the occasions in your life when to present yourself really well is of the utmost importance. So — bear in mind the following points:

1 Dress well, but don't overdo it — remember you're not going to a party! If you know you look 'good' in your clothes, you will feel 'good' and gain confidence.

2 Remember the job you're hoping to get and wear make-up and a hair-style that is appropriate for it.

3 When you meet the person who is going to interview you — do greet them with a smile and a handshake (which should not be of the 'rugby player crunch' or the 'limp lettuce' variety!). The smile will help to make you feel more relaxed if you're feeling nervous, because your facial muscles will lose their tenseness.

4 When you are asked to sit down, try to sit comfortably in your chair without slumping or sagging in it. The minute you slump — you lose authority.

5 Do answer questions as fully as possible. You may be feeling nervous and shy but that is no excuse to answer with a mere 'yes' or 'no'. Remember you are there to get a job and you must contribute as much as possible to the interview. Be courteous and pleasant at all times — never 'off-hand', which is usually interpreted as rudeness, even if that wasn't the intention. Finally, do not underestimate yourself. Be confident and enthusiastic and you will impress. Good luck!

Task 1

List all the things you would want to know at an interview.

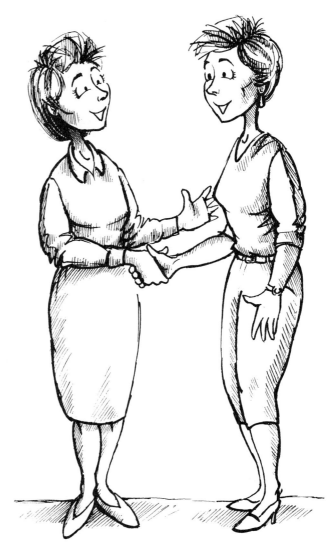

Task 2

Most candidates are invited at some time or other by the interviewer to 'tell me something about yourself'. Spend a short time talking to another member of the group and then say what he or she has told you about himself or herself.

Assignment 8: Working on a liner

Read the following passage carefully.

Working on a liner is many a beauty therapist's ambition. There are drawbacks, however. The reality is that you are away from friends and family, for months at a time, confined by the ship. You have only limited space to work in and may suffer some degee of seasickness initially. The living quarters are cramped and you will have to share a cabin and shower room with other members of the female staff. There are usually separate facilities for the crew, because mixing with the passengers is prohibited. You are employed to look after the passengers, so they must always come first. You are under the authority of the ship's captain and your shore leave is at his discretion. You must abide by the conditions in your contract, or you will be sent home.

All the ships want therapists with experience and massage is important. You must also be single. Obviously working on a liner does give you the opportunity to visit countries that you may not otherwise have the chance to, and the experience can be very rewarding. The basic wage may appear low, but all your living expenses are paid for. The

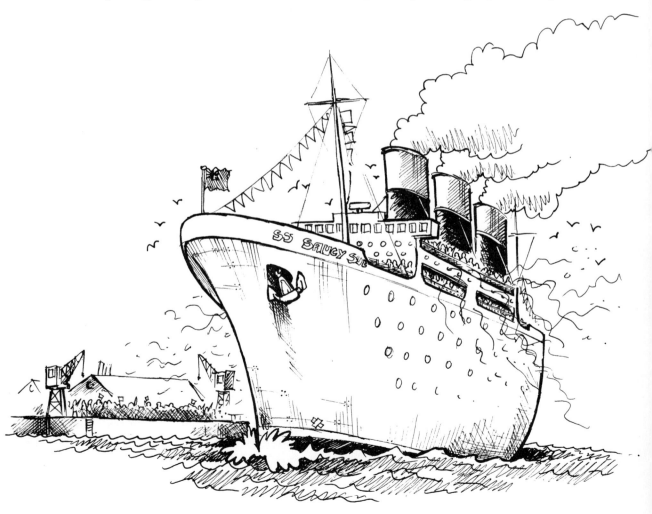

commission and tips can make it quite a substantial income, the money you get though, does depend very much on you. How much you put into your work, and how you treat the clients; acting politely and pleasantly all affect your income. There is a lot of competition for the jobs on the ships, and so a very high standard of work is demanded. Good physical health, professionalism and a groomed appearance also count.

From 'Careers in Beauty Therapy' by Louise Kelly. *Health and Beauty Salon* (August/September 1985).

Task 1

Answer the following questions:
1 Of all the drawbacks mentioned in the passage, which one would *you* consider to be the greatest and why?
2 What are the chief attractions of such a job?
3 Why do you think a low basic wage is acceptable in such a job?
4 The passage states: 'There is a lot of competition for the jobs on the ship.' What do you consider are the qualities needed for such work?

Task 2

Imagine that you are giving a commentary from one of the following:
(a) The quayside
(b) The railway station
(c) The departure lounge at an airport
as a celebrity of your own choice is about to depart. Describe the scene as vividly as possible in script form.

Task 3

Write a letter to:
Justine Smythe,
Cruising Beauty Ltd.,
10, Ocean Way,
Southampton,
Hants. SO4 WS1.
requesting information about 'Working on a Liner'.

Assignment 9: The demonstration

A brochure from a well-known firm of make-up and beauty products arrives in the post one day. It gives details of a new range of products called 'The Atlantis Range' and offers tempting discounts on purchases made as a result of a demonstration by one of their make-up and beauty experts in your own salon.

You are interested in this offer.

Task 1

Write a letter to:
    Martyne Products Ltd.,
    29, Mansion Gardens,
    Hatton,
    London. W1. 4LS.
inviting their demonstrator to visit your salon.

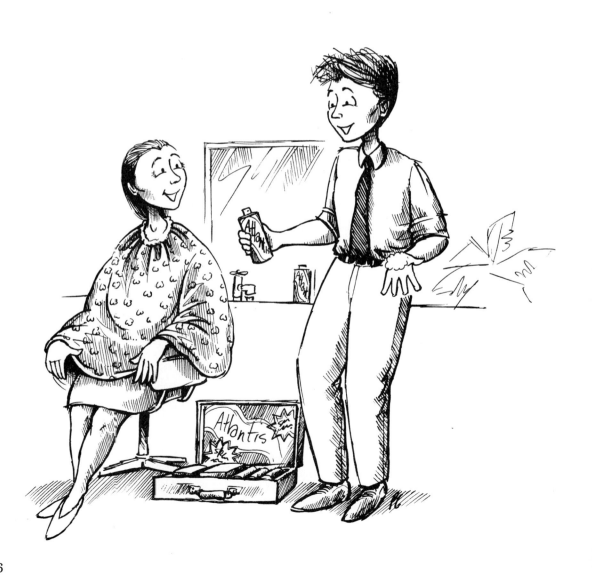

Task 2

As a result of the demonstration, you decide to stock a limited amount of 'The Atlantis Range' for a trial period of 6 months. Write the appropriate letter to Ms. A. Green, of Martyne Products Ltd., confirming the arrangement.

Task 3

Write a memo to the owner of your salon, giving details of the decision.

Task 4

At the end of 6 months, you have only sold one bottle of 'The Atlantis Range' moisturising lotion, so you decide to ask a representative from Martyne's Products to come and remove the remainder of the stock.

Paying particular attention to 'tone', write the appropriate letter to him or her.

Guide-lines on graphics

Apart from the quality of work produced in any salon, much of the success of the establishment depends on the way it presents itself to the general public, and the image it portrays through the appearance of its staff, and the design of the furnishings, lighting and general decoration. Equally important is the 'marketing' of the establishment through advertisements, appointment cards, brochures, tariffs, notices, and headed paper. Remember — you look at the appearance of the salon first and probably read the price list before you decide

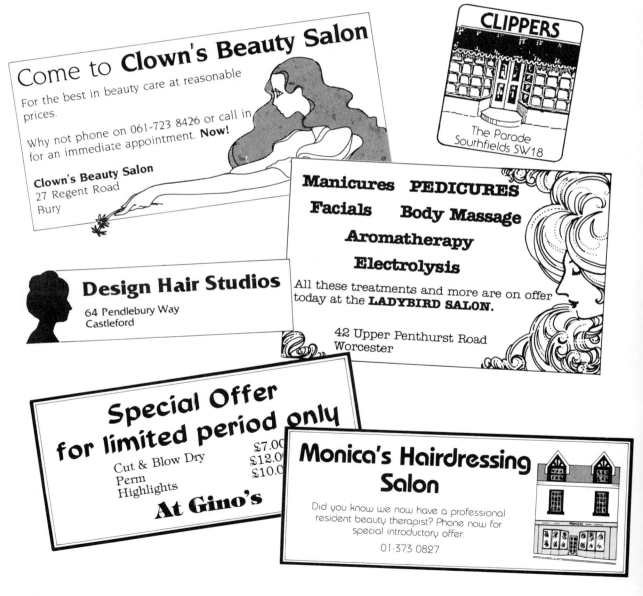

to go in! The following points are important:

1 Anything that is graphically represented must be easily seen and understood, so it must be *eye-catching*, *readable* and *clear*.
2 Beware of being too fussy. The best designs are often the simplest.

The following equipment and techniques will help you to achieve a degree of professionalism.

Dry brush stencilling

This is a very effective and simple method of lettering which has the great advantage of being relatively cheap. It involves using a special brush which is moistened very slightly on a damp felt pad and then worked into colour until it is nearly dry. It is then rubbed over the appropriate stencil.

Pen stencilling

This is a sophisticated technique involving the use of special pens, templates and stencils. The equipment is expensive, but would be a worthwhile investment if it is going to be used extensively.

Dry transfer printing

This is a very popular form of printing using letters and symbols which are printed on to paper by simply rubbing them off with the

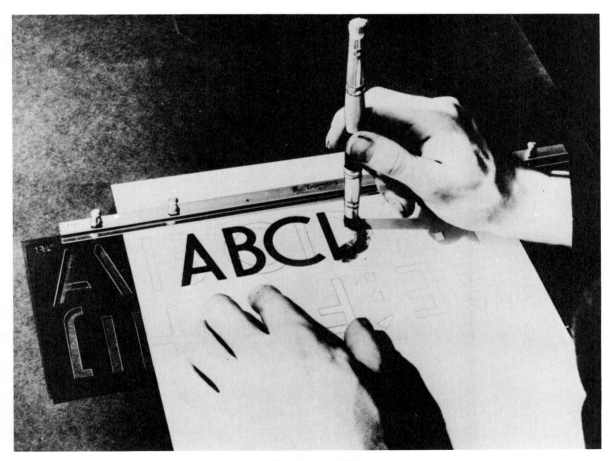

Dry brush stencilling

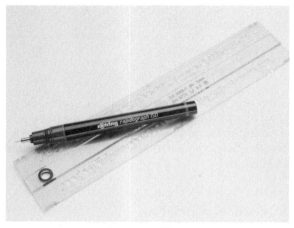

Pen stencilling

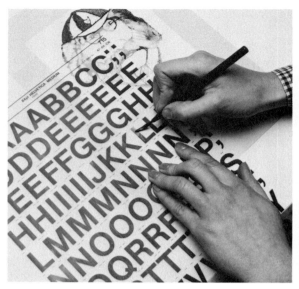

Dry transfer printing

rounded head of a pen or pencil. The result is extremely professional, and a tremendous variety of letters and symbols are available.

All these aids should be very familar to art departments or graphics units of schools or colleges. However, information and equipment for Dry Brush Stencilling is available from The Econasign Co. Ltd., 31, Britton Street, London. EC1M 5NQ.

Pen stencilling equipment is produced by firms such as Rotring and Staedler, and may be obtained from any good stationer or art supplier.

Dry transfer sheets produced by firms such as Letraset similarly may be obtained from any good stationer or art supplier.

Assignment 10: The fashion show

The situation

You are approaching the end of your Hairdressing and Beauty course, and it has been decided that you will combine with the Art and Design students in producing a fashion show at the end of term, with proceeds to be given to a charity.

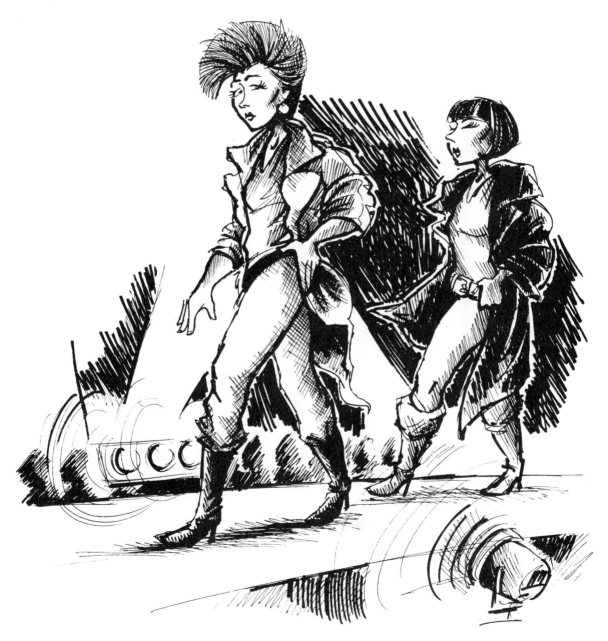

Task 1

Make a list of all the factors that must be considered.

Task 2

Lighting is obviously on your list. Write a letter to:
    Disco Lighting, Ltd.,
    5 Shotton Street,
    Birmingham
telling them about your Fashion Show and enquiring about their services. You may feel like inviting a representative of the firm to come and talk to you.

Task 3

Design a poster advertising the event from the Hairdressing and Beauty angle.

Task 4

Design the invitation.

Task 5

Write an account of the scene in the dressing room 10 minutes before the show opens, trying to capture the feeling of excitement.

Task 6

Write a letter to your local newspaper after the very successful event, thanking the public for their support.

Assignment 11: The hair

Please read the following passage carefully:

The hair

Nestlé's wonder machine for 'perming', although invented in 1906, only really hit the masses in the 1920s, changing the manes of nations. In London Eugène claimed to be the 'ablest and most renowned permanent Hair Waver of Paris & London' ... the Mason Pearson hairbrush was 'enjoyed by all' ... and Inecto-Rapid was 'used by ROYALTY, endorsed by 5,000 leading hairdressers' and 'permanently restored colour to Grey Hair in 15 minutes'. *Vogue* warned: 'Ill-kept hair spoils all possibilities of good looks and smartness.' By 1929 the shingle had succeeded the bob and the Eton crop was soon to come. With the 1930s came a 'new sense of individuality'. 'Curls must never appear untidy and so, to hold them in perfect control, some of the smartest women are adding to their coiffures decorative details that are practical, smart and becoming.' You could keep your hair in 'perfect order' with a Lady Jayne Slumbernet and 'science' discovered a way to bring back colour and gloss to faded hair 'by natural methods' — the only method 'endorsed by the Press'. But just in case that didn't work you could buy a bobbed head-dress for eighteen guineas. There was increasing interest in hair care and *Vogue* advised 'a good shampoo every two, or perhaps three weeks'. In the 1940s hair fashion was dictated by the war: girls working in factories had to wear turbans and snoods to stop their long hair getting into the machinery and servicewomen had to wear their hair above the collar. *Vogue* asked: 'Why does that shoulder-mane seem so out of date?' With the 1950s the teenagers took over, first with the ponytail, later with the loose hair cult and the Carita sisters in Paris made the first fashion wigs — to match Givenchy dresses. The accent was on *you*. André Bernard's 'creations moulded to suit your individual charms': French's creations 'for you alone': Riché's 'short-styled softly waving coiffure — the fashion follows you'. The wig boom began in 1960. Harrods — like other big stores — opened a wig counter and by the end of the decade the State was supplying human hair on the N.H.S. In 1963 Vidal Sassoon created his revolutionary new haircut — hard, architectural, thick cropped bob — and later came Jean Shrimpton's 'tiger mane', pre-Raphaelite 'ripple waves' and the first 'afro' styles. With the 1970s hair health became a fetish: henna brightened the colour, added shine and weight. 'With less backcombing, less lacquer, more brushing, more shine, there's a new deal in hair health.'

From: Vogue Body and Beauty Book, Bronwen Meredith (Allen Lane, Penguin Books Ltd. 1977).

Task 1

Now answer the following questions:
1 How long did it take for Nestlé's 'perming machine' to become popular?
2 What did the Inecto-Rapid treatment claim to do?
3 What hair styles were popular at the end of the 1920s and the beginning of the 1930s?
4 What 5 words tell you that in the 1930s a very *neat* hairstyle was fashionable?
5 What could you buy to keep your hair tidy while you were sleeping?
6 What was 'a bobbed head-dress'? How much would it have cost you? Why might you have bought it?
7 How often should women shampoo their hair according to Vogue?
8 What influenced hair fashion in the 1940s?
9 When did the cult of the teenagers begin?
10 Why do you think Vidal Sassoon's new hairstyle creation was described as 'revolutionary'?
11 Who was Jean Shrimpton and how did her hair-styles differ from the typical Vidal Sassoon 'look'?
12 What was the great influence of the 1970s?

Task 2

What do you understand by the following:
1 The 'shingle'.

33

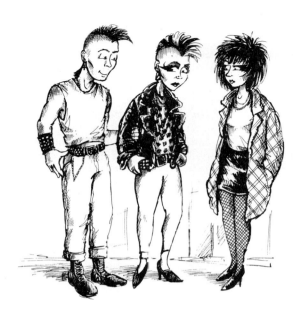

2 The 'bob'.
3 The 'Eton crop'.
4 'Snoods'.
5 'Fetish'.

Task 3

Add your own ending to the passage by writing a paragraph on the influences and styles of the 1980s.

Assignment 12: The beauty course

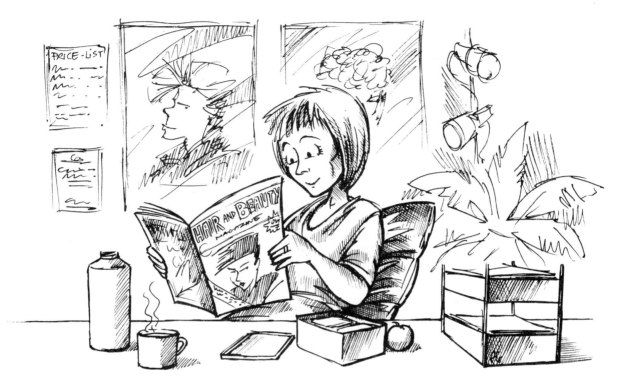

The situation

You are looking through a *Hair and Beauty* magazine one lunch hour when you see the following advertisement:

> Extend your experience and improve your career opportunities. Enrol now for one of our exciting one-day courses on Stage and Film Make-up run by leading specialists from the theatre and the film industry. Full details from:
> "The Back-Stage" School,
> 31 Grease-Paint Gardens,
> Soho,
> London W1

Task 1

Most advertisements of this sort carry a 'bait'. What is the bait in this one?

Rewrite the opening line of this advertisement:
(a) To appeal to the reader who is lonely.
(b) To suggest an interesting alternative to the usual weekend.

Task 2

Write a letter to 'The Back-Stage' School, asking for details.

Task 3

What essential information would be given in the details?

Task 4

You are impressed by the details 'The Back-Stage' School send back to you. Write a letter enrolling for one of their courses.

Assignment 13: New stationery for the salon

You are idly reading a copy of *Hair and Beauty* during a coffee break one morning in the salon, when you notice the following advertisement:

Give Your Salon A New Image

Top quality stationery at very low prices.

Order your headed paper, price lists, and appointment cards etc. now, and take advantage of our special introductory price offer.

Write for catalogue and price list to:
Top Flight Stationery Supplies Ltd.,
9 Hoskin Lane, London S.E.4.

Task 1

Write to Top Flight Stationery Supplies Ltd. for a catalogue and price list.

Task 2

Top Flight Stationery Supplies Ltd. send you the catalogue but not the price list. Write an appropriate letter of complaint.

Task 3

You are secretary to the sales manager of Top Flight Stationery Supplies Ltd. Write a letter of apology to the Mayfair Salon, 15, High Street, Chesbury, Gloucestershire CH5 3GL to accompany the price list you will send.

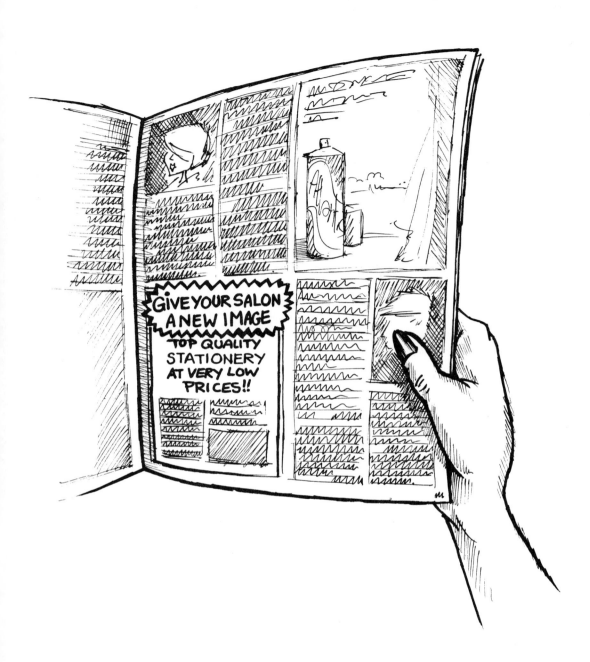

Assignment 14: The Dimchester festival competition

You work in a very successful salon in a large market town in the south-west. Each year the town organises a festival, and apart from the usual fair and music and drama, all sorts of local competitions are held. This year the festival committee has written to you inviting you to organise a hairdressing competition, drawing on students from the nearby technical college and young apprentices from the local salons.

Task 1

Design the entry form for the competition, bearing in mind that there may be different categories of entry.

Task 2

You obviously need a hall in which to stage the competition. Write to the local education authority asking whether St. Cuthbert's School Hall may be used for the competition on a particular date, and enquiring what the charge will be.

Task 3

Write an advertisement for the competition to be placed in the local newspaper.

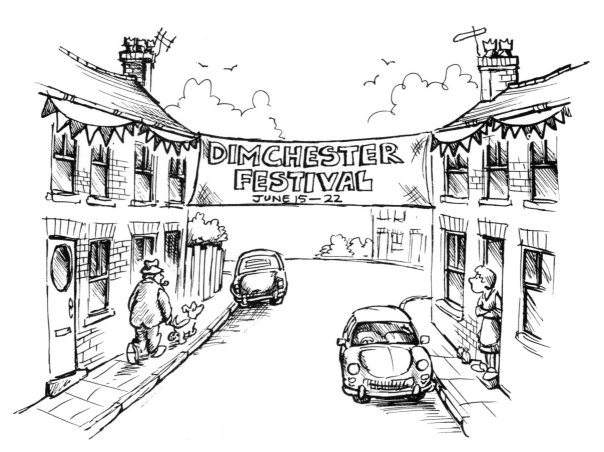

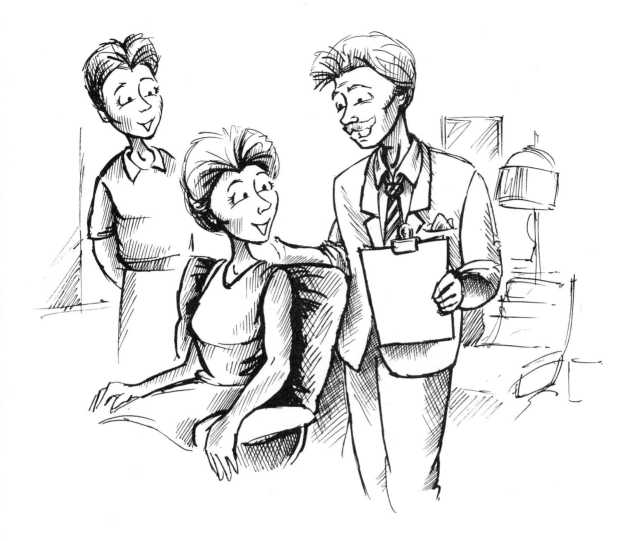

Task 4

Write an invitation to a well-known hair-dresser, asking him or her to act as judge.

Task 5

Write a thank-you letter to him or her after the event.

Guide-lines on preparing a short talk

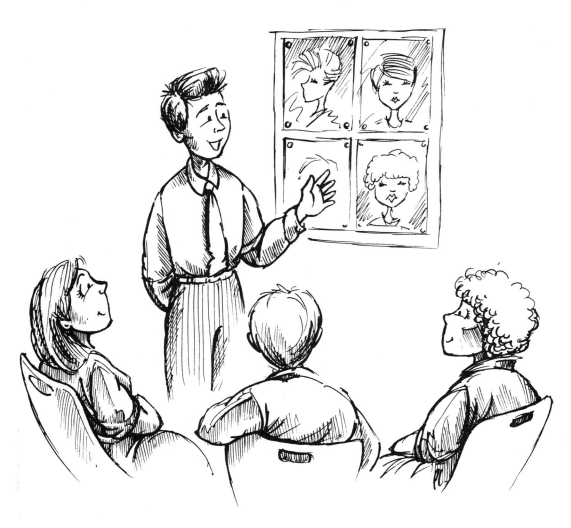

1 When you know the subject of your talk, write down all ideas, words and phrases that are relevant to the subject.
2 You should now have a very random and disjointed list. Arrange it into logical order.
3 The next step is to sort the order into sections. What are you going to talk about first? How are you going to develop it? How are you going to finish?
4 Your talk is beginning to take shape! Now, plan the *introduction*. This is very impor-

tant. You must make your listeners want to listen to you and to feel that what you have to say is going to be worth while and enjoyable. The mood is usually established in the introduction, so plan it carefully.
5 Write the whole talk out in full, read it out loud and make any alterations that you feel may be necessary. The actual writing out will help to commit the content and the shape of the talk to your memory. Now, with equal care, plan the *conclusion*, which should bring your talk to a definite and

memorable end. Avoid phrases like 'and that's about it, really!'

6 Consider the visual aids you will need for your talk: posters, pictures, photographs, diagrams, etc. Please make sure they are big enough to be seen and that the diagrams are bold (you can easily check your visual aids in advance). If you are using small photographs, mount them on to card and show them under your control at the appropriate time during your talk, or invite your audience to come and look at them afterwards. Never pass photos or objects round while you are actually talking, otherwise your audience will stop listening to you!

7 If you are using any technical equipment, make quite sure that you know how it works! Prepare slides, etc., well in advance so that you show them the right way round and in the correct order!

8 Now transfer your talk in heading form only on to small pieces of card called 'Cue Cards'. These are to remind you of what you are going to say. Avoid trying to memorise the whole thing word for word, but do practise in front of a friend or friends if possible. If not, use a mirror. Preparation is very important indeed.

9 Stand comfortably, relax and look at your audience. And finally

10 Talk *to* your audience, never *at* them. Smile at them — you have something to say which they will enjoy — share it with them. If you have prepared well, you will be confident. If you are confident, you will be enthusiastic, and if you have the combination of confidence and enthusiasm, the chances are that you will be very good indeed!

Guide-lines on preparing a demonstration

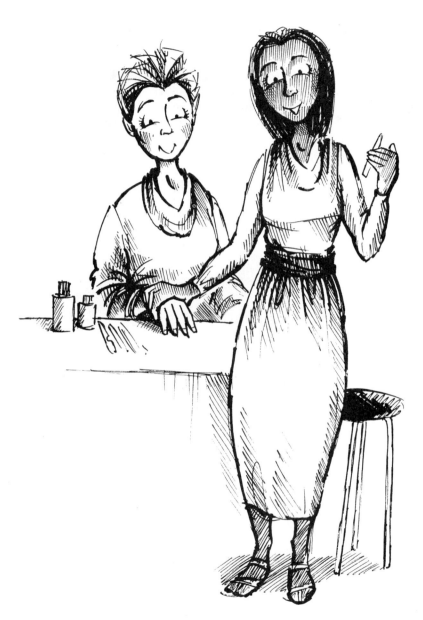

1 Make a list of all the pieces of equipment you will need, and make quite sure that they are ready for use (i.e. clean, and in working order).

2 Lay your equipment out in an orderly way so that you don't have to search (or scrabble around in a bag!) for a particular piece of equipment.

3 Plan the introduction to your demonstration (see Note 4 of 'Preparing a short talk').

4 Now to the demonstration itself. Guide your listeners through it step by step, avoiding

long silent gaps as you demonstrate a particular skill. It's very important to rehearse your demonstration so that you know when the gaps are likely to occur and can prepare accordingly.

5 Don't panic if something goes wrong; audiences are amazingly sympathetic, especially if you take them into your confidence and explain how and why the mistake occurred and how you would correct it.

6 Plan the conclusion of your demonstration and remember that people love to see clearly the end product, whatever it might be. You can always invite your audience to take a closer look.

7 Note 10 of 'Preparing a short talk' applies equally here — read it carefully.

Assignment 15: The careers evening

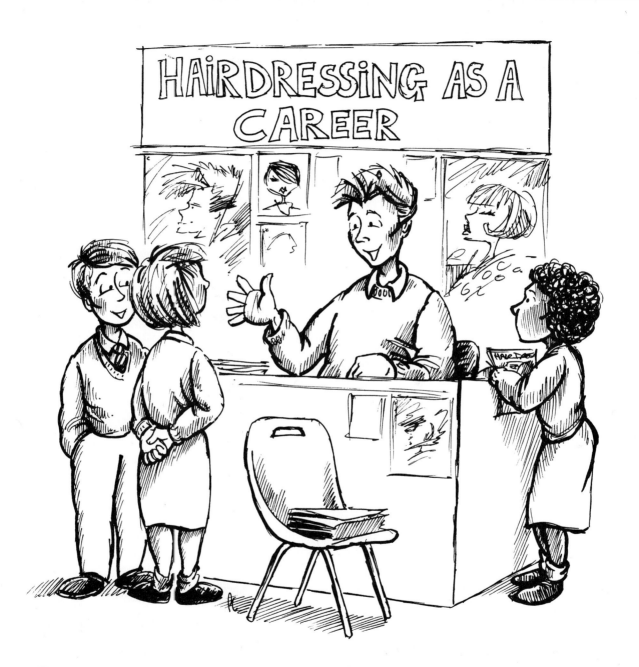

The situation

Your salon has been approached by a local school and asked to attend a 'Careers Convention'. A large number of pupils in the school 'have expressed an interest in hairdressing and beauty care as a career and you have been allocated a classroom for your exhibition.

Task

Choose one of the following:

1 Using a model and any aids you think are necessary, prepare and give a demonstration of a skill learned in your course to interest a group of school-leavers.

2 Prepare and give a talk to a group of school-leavers on 'Hairdressing (or Beauty Care) as a Career'.

Assignment 16: Barriers

The following letter appeared in a local paper recently.

Sir,

I cannot understand what is happening to young people today. When I was shopping in the High Street the other day I noticed a group sitting on the benches and seats in 'The Square'. Some of them had their heads completely shaved, others had their heads shaved at the sides, but with the hair on the top of their heads standing up on end, giving the impression of people undergoing severe electric shocks. Some had multi-coloured hair and wore bizarre make-up, and others were dressed completely in black and white with ear-rings and jewellery very much in evidence. It was extremely difficult to tell the sexes apart, and I'm quite certain I would never have been allowed to look like that in my young day. The language, I could not help but over-hear, was quite appalling. I am quite used to bad language, having served as a soldier in World War II but I never thought I would hear such obscenities coming from the lips of such young people. The benches and seats they were sitting on were covered with writing, some of which was misspelt and the whole area seemed to be littered with cans, paper and general rubbish, although there were litter-bins nearby. What has happened to this once great nation?

Signed: John Bull

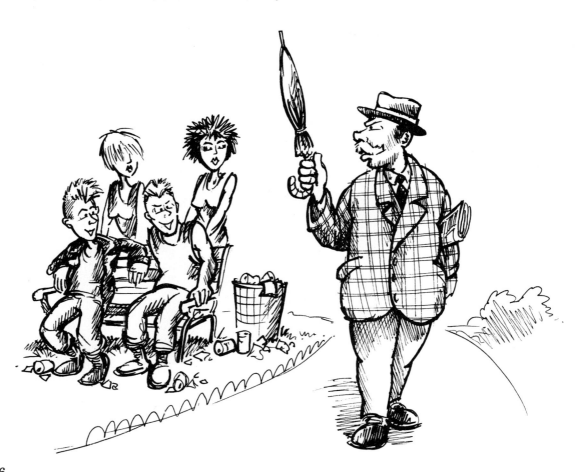

Task 1

Answer the following:
1 The writer is probably
  (a) over 60 years of age
  (b) between 45 and 55 years of age
  (c) under 55 years of age.
2 The writer is
  (a) furious
  (b) bewildered
  (c) appalled
  by the appearance of the young people.
3 The make-up worn by some of the young people was
  (a) fantastic
  (b) conventional
  (c) colourful.
4 Another word to describe the language overheard by the writer would be
  (a) vulgar
  (b) strident
  (c) indecent.
5 The writing on the seats and benches is known as
  (a) racist
  (b) graffiti
  (c) sexist.

6 The last sentence shows that the writer is
  (a) proud
  (b) prejudiced
  (c) patriotic.

Task 2

Which areas of the letter do you think are legitimate areas for concern? Which areas reveal the writer's prejudices? What is the main 'barrier' revealed by the letter?

Task 3

Make a list of all the barriers you can think of in our society today.

Task 4

As a group (or groups) discuss them and suggest ways in which they can be broken down.

Task 5

Imagine *you* are writing to the newspaper in the year 2000. Describe the scene in 'The Square' then.

Assignment 17: Trouble in the salon

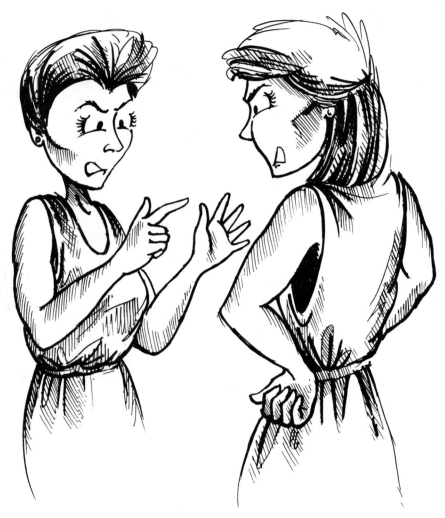

The situation

You have recently started work as a young assistant in Simone's Salon, which enjoys the reputation of being well organised and friendly, offering a high class service for a reasonable price. Simone (whose real name is Sue) is the owner/manager. She took out a heavy bank loan four years ago to set up the business and, although she had an initial struggle to get established, she feels that now her business is successful, and that she should

soon have reduced her bank loan considerably. She has 4 assistants:

1 Derek — an excellent hairdresser who has been with her since the salon opened. He has real flair and is very popular with the customers.

2 Jill, who is a hard-working YTS trainee, hoping to be offered a job at the end of her training course.

3 Debbie, who started work in the salon 2 years ago when she left college. She is quite competent as a hairdresser, and is popular

among the older customers, who enjoy chatting to her. She does, however, tend to be rather slapdash and inclined to forget to take customers out of the drier when she gets involved in a conversation.

4 Yvonne, the beautician, who is inclined to think she is rather superior to the others, except Derek, whose talent she admires. Although she is excellent at her job, she is not very popular with the others and one day when Sue (Simone) is away ill a 'spot of bother' occurs.

Task 1

As a group, adopt the roles of the main characters (note that I have deliberately left the customers for you to create) and devise the 'spot of trouble' which occurs one day when the manager/owner is away ill.

Task 2

As an individual, write to Sue during her illness to tell her about the trouble, and how it was resolved.

Task 3

Imagine that you are Sue, and write a letter to a friend you haven't seen since he/she went abroad 4 years ago, telling him/her about your business venture.

Assignment 18: The fancy dress party

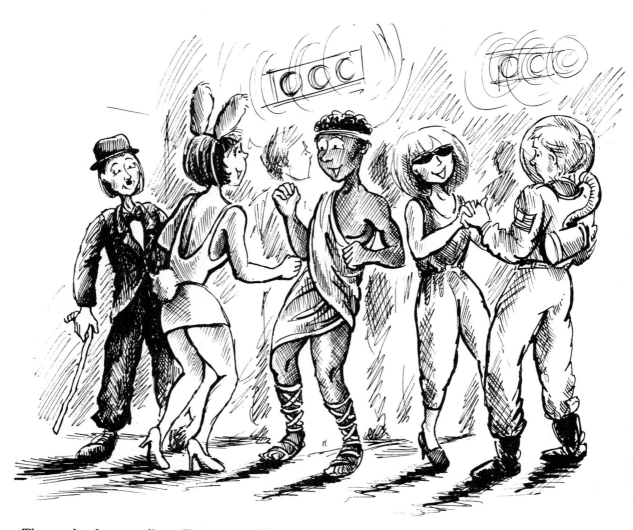

The end of your first Term at college is approaching and everyone is looking forward to Christmas. Someone in the group suggests having a fancy dress party to celebrate.

Task 1

As an individual, decide on a 'theme' for the party and produce
(a) an appropriate invitation and poster
(b) a letter to
'King Kong' Fancy Dress Hire,
7, High Street,
Cloudsville,
Leicestershire L13 CL4
asking them if they can supply appropriate costumes and a price list.

Task 2

As a group (or groups) choose one of the themes and design the hair-styles and make-up, using sketches, and models if possible. Notes and an oral explanation should accompany the sketches and models.

Assignment 19: Accident in the salon

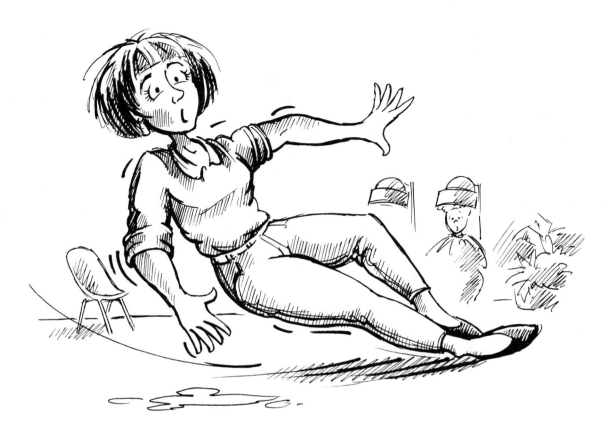

You are working in the salon one day when a colleague slips on some spilt setting lotion. She cuts her leg, which subsequently needs 4 stitches, and sprains her ankle rather badly.

Task 1

Write out a full report of the accident for the insurance company giving
(a) date
(b) time
(c) place
(d) your own account of what happened, using a sketch plan if necessary
(e) details of first-aid given
(f) names and addresses of two witnesses who can be contacted if necessary.

Task 2

As a result of the accident, the manager of the salon suspects that the floor covering in the shampooing area should be changed, and asks you to do some research into floor coverings and surfaces for use in areas where spillages are likely to occur. This necessitates looking at trade literature and possibly writing away for information. You should present your research in the form of a short report to give to your manager.

Guide-lines on writing a short report

Don't be 'put off' by the word report. Remember that, quite simply, a report is written to someone, by someone, about something. It should be as simple and straightforward as possible, and because it is the result of careful investigation, it must be arranged in some sort of logical order. It must be readable and therefore it should be attractively presented. Remember that if you find it boring to write, it will probably be boring to read!

A report should be arranged as follows:

1 Title page — title of subject and name of author.
2 Aim — a brief, clear statement of the purpose of the report.
3 Contents — a list of the sections of the report.
4 The main body of the report arranged in logical order.
5 Conclusion.
6 Recommendations.
7 Bibliography — a list of books and publications used.
8 Appendices — any tables, graphs and diagrams which are 'extra' and not easily inserted into the main text should be placed in this section at the end of the report.

Assignment 20: The new solarium

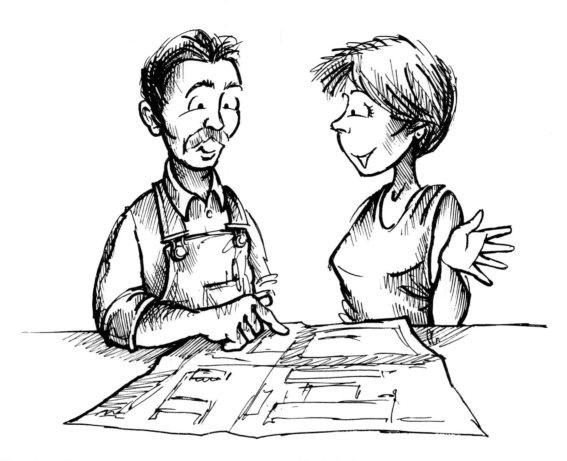

The situation

You are working in a small, but very successful, hairdressing salon, and for some time now you have thought that business would improve even more if some additional services could be offered. There is a room at the back of the salon which you feel could be converted fairly easily into a solarium with facilities for beauty therapy and you mention this to the owner. She thinks it an excellent idea and asks you to 'get something down on paper' . . .

Task 1

Draw a plan of the room, showing the proposed layout of the new equipment.

Task 2

Add notes to the drawing to indicate decoration (paint colour, wallpaper, floor covering, furnishing fabrics, etc.).

Task 3

Write a letter to the owner (who is at home recovering from a minor operation) to accompany the drawing and notes, hoping that the owner will approve of all you've done.

Task 4

The owner is delighted and asks you to write to a local (imaginary) builder, inviting him to visit the salon and give an approximate estimate for carrying out the decorating and any alterations that are needed.

Task 5

Write a memo to the owner (who is now back at work), reminding her that the builder will be starting work on the new solarium next week.

Assignment 21: Consumer report

The situation

You have just started a Hairdressing and Beauty course at your local College of Further Education and find that your services as a hairdresser are increasingly in demand amongst your friends. Your family suggest that you buy your own blow dryer, but there are now so many on the market it is difficult to know which one to choose.

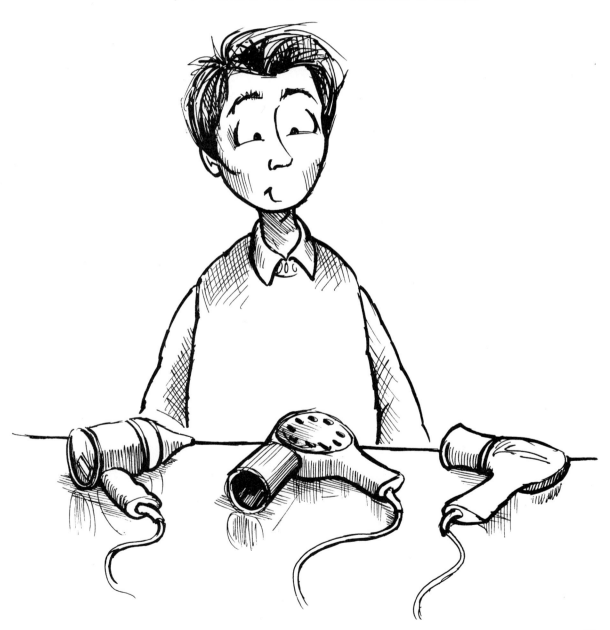

Task 1

Select 6 blow dryers currently available and, bearing in mind such things as cost, ease of use, design, and your particular needs, select one of them as your 'best buy'.

Task 2

Present your findings in the form of a short report, justifying your choice.

Task 3

Write a set of clear instructions, describing the process of connecting a plug to your blow dryer, using a diagram to help you.

Assignment 22: The college play

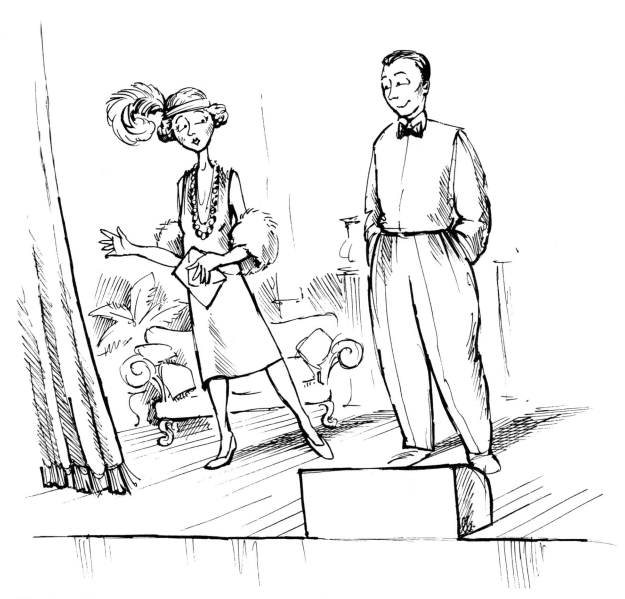

The situation

The Speech and Drama Department of your college are currently involved in their production of 'The Boy Friend', and they have called upon the services of the Hairdressing and Beauty Department to design the hair and make-up for the production.

Task 1

Obviously you have got to do a little research first. So, using the resources of your college library find out the answers to the following questions.
1 Who wrote 'The Boy Friend'?

2 Is the play
   (a) a tragedy?
   (b) a comedy?
   (c) a 'musical'?
   (d) a 'farce'?
   (e) a 'straight' play?
3 In what era is the play set?
4 Describe very briefly the main characters.

Task 2

Prepare a set of notes with sketches, setting out your ideas for the hair and make-up designs to give to the producer.

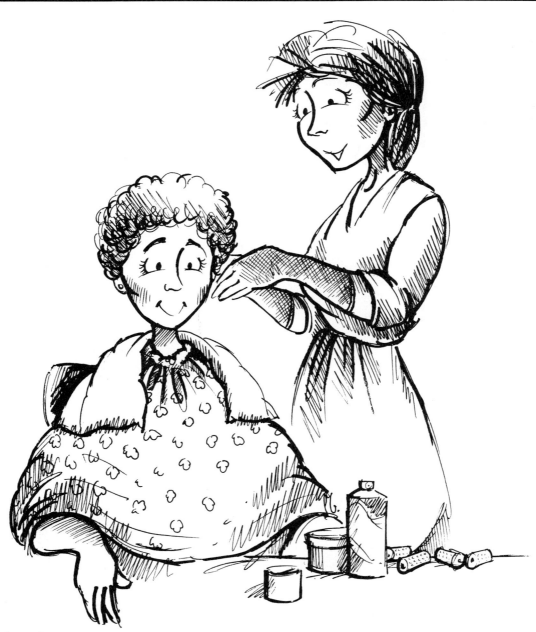

The situation

Read the following very carefully:

Wash the hair very thoroughly and rub it brisk-ly with a towel to remove the excess moisture. Next, part the hair so that it is divided into 9 equal parts and wet thoroughly with the solution. Curl appropriate strands of hair on to the correct curlers and damp down again with the lotion. Leave your client for 5 to 15 minutes and check from time to time to see how tight the curl is. Now spray water over the head and thoroughly wash away the solution. Pat the mixture that makes

59

the curl stay in shape over the head, and then spray water over the head again. Take out the curlers and set the hair as you would normally do.

P.S. Be careful, when you are treating bleached and tinted hair, to mix the lotion and the water into equal parts.

Task 1

Give a title to the above and rewrite it in the form of a set of 12 simple instructions.

Task 2

Choose one instruction and describe carefully how you would do it.

Task 3

Think of a client who has received the above treatment from you. Describe him/her and write of something that went wrong — real or imaginery.

Assignment 24: The young beautician

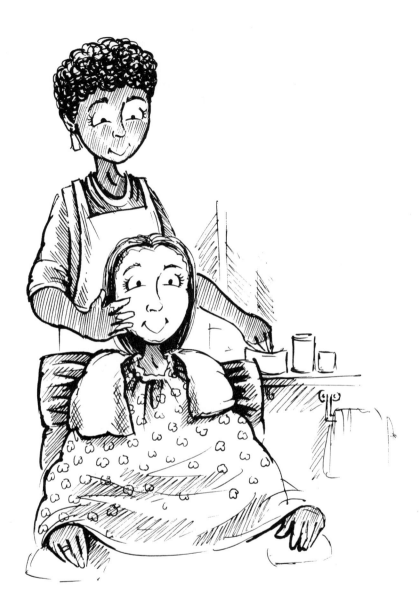

Read the following carefully:

'Young beauticians may find some prejudice against them because of their youth, as some employers do feel that their clients, mainly older women, prefer to have treatment from someone mature who understands their particular problems. On the other hand the teenager seeking a lesson in make-up, the fashion model needing help with a figure problem or the bride wanting a very special facial just before her wedding will enjoy meeting a beauty expert who is young too. The essential qualities for a successful beautician of any age is a warm sympathetic personality, and a sincere interest in the problems of her clients. At the moment young beauticians are working in salons attached to department stores, international hotels and on board ship. Over the last few years great numbers of women have come to depend on the skill of the hairdresser; it is only a matter of time before they begin to demand the same kind of expert help for their faces and figures too. The trained beautician will then be in great demand to staff and manage new salons all over the country.'

From *Hairdressing and Beauty Culture*, a picture career book by Patrick Ward (Lutterworth Press, 1963).

Task

Answer the following questions:

1 Why would some employers be unwilling to offer a job to a young beautician?
2 Name 2 groups of young people who would enjoy meeting a young beauty expert.
3 What are the special qualities needed by a successful beautician?
4 Name 3 areas in which a beautician may find employment.
5 Choose one area of work from your answer to number 4 in which you would seek employment. Give reasons for your choice.
6 Which sentences show that this extract was written 20 years ago.
7 How has the situation changed now?
8 Apart from giving advice on make-up, what else would a beautician advise on?
9 Which part of a beautician's work are you particularly interested in? Why?
10 Describe a typical morning in a beautician's salon.

Assignment 25: *Easter in Paris*

It is a particularly dreary and grey day at the end of January. The delights of Christmas have now disappeared into the past, but the spring is still far away into the future. One cold, wet lunch hour you happen to glance into a travel agent's window and see a large poster advertising an Easter Break in Paris. It looks very attractive and you decide to investigate further. You enter the travel agent's and pick up the appropriate brochure.

Task 1

Study the information given overleaf and answer the following questions:

1 If you decided to take your own car with you how long would it take you (approximately) to cross the Channel by hovercraft and drive to Paris?
2 You decide to spend four nights in Paris, staying in an hotel described in the brochure as 'budget tourist grade' and your rooms (there are 4 of you) have a bathroom or shower adjoining. How much would the basic cost be for each of you?
3 If you went by train and took an overnight boat:

(a) when would you leave London?
(b) when would you arrive in Paris?

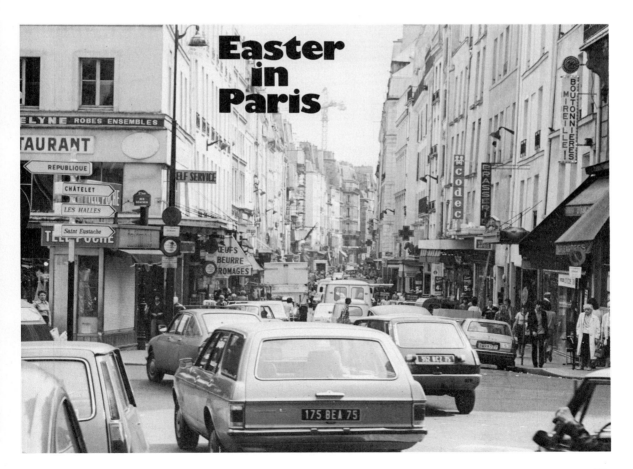

(c) how long would the journey take from London to Paris?

4 If you decided to travel by air from Gatwick or Heathrow, at which Paris airport would you land?

5 Name another airport in Paris.

6 What is the tour number of the cheapest Easter break?
What is the tour number of the most expensive?

Task 2

Using the facilities of your college library or other sources, write a brief paragraph on each of the following:
1 Charles de Gaulle.
2 Les Bateaux Mouches.
3 Le Centre Pompidou.
4 The Eiffel Tower.
5 The 'Left Bank'.

Easter and all the Bank Holidays for 1985		EASTER				BANK HOLIDAYS (May, Spring & August)			
		depart Thursday or Friday 4 NIGHTS		depart Friday 3 NIGHTS		depart Friday 3 NIGHTS		depart Saturday 2 NIGHTS	
Tour No	Travel Route	PH1 PH2 PH3 PH4	PH1 PH2 PH3 PH4	PH1 PH2 PH3 PH4	PH1 PH2 PH3 PH4
PCE	**Paris Coach Express**	not available	63 72 79 —	61 70 77 —	not available
BR1	**Rail** - ship or hovercraft - day services	74 85 94 110	66 76 83 95	64 74 81 93	59 66 71 78
EXO	**Rail** - ship overnight service (3 nights hotel)	68 79 89 99	not available	not available	not available
PAE	**Paris Air Express**	not available	79 88 94 104	77 86 92 102	not available
BCA	**British Caledonian** (Gatwick)	106 118 125 142	100 109 114 127	98 107 112 125	92 98 102 110
BAF	**British Airways or Air France** (Heathrow)	111 123 130 147	105 114 119 132	103 112 117 130	97 103 107 115
TYC	**Take your own car** (each of 4 persons)	64 76 84 100	58 67 73 85	56 65 71 83	50 56 60 68

Hotel grade explanation:
(For details see pages 6/7)
PH1: Budget tourist grade without bath/shower
PH2: Budget tourist grade with bath/shower
PH3: Tourist grade with bath/shower
PH4: Higher grade with bath/shower

Single rooms: PH1 £4; PH2 £6; PH3 £8; PH4 £10 per night.
Twin rooms: £1 per person per night.

Take your own car is based on 4 persons per car. Supplements for only 3 in a car £6 each and only 2 in a car £16 each. August Bank Holiday supplement £22 per car.
Prices are in £'s per person in double room (large bed) according to Hotel grade and travel route selected.

ITINERARY: Rail/ship overnight services (Easter only)

Depart London late Thursday evening (approx. 9p.m.) via Newhaven - Dieppe. Ship crossing approx. 4 hrs. Arrive Paris, St. Lazare approx. 7a.m. Friday morning. Coach transfer to hotel and breakfast. Three nights hotel. Return similar timings on Monday evening arriving London Tuesday morning.

ITINERARY: Scheduled Air from Gatwick or Heathrow

Depart Gatwick or Heathrow mid-morning or afternoon to Paris, Charles de Gaulle airport (1 hr.). Make your own way from the airport by bus or train (27 Frs.) to central Paris and taxi or Metro to your hotel. Return on afternoon or evening services.

ITINERARY: Take your own car

Depart Dover at a time to suit your driving time from your hometown. Please state clearly on the Booking Form your earliest preferred departure from and latest return to Dover. Cross channel by hovercraft to Calais or Boulogne and approx. 3½ hrs. drive into Paris. Parking cannot be guaranteed.

ITINERARY: Paris-Air Express

Depart Gatwick, early afternoon Friday by Dan-Air 1-11 Jet for Beauvais (40 mins.) and express coach direct from the airport to your hotel arriving early evening. Three nights hotel. Early afternoon departure on Monday from central Paris terminal arriving Gatwick late afternoon.

ITINERARY: Daytime rail/ship or hovercraft

Depart London mid-morning or midday by train (with reserved seats) for Dover. Ship crossing approx. 1½ hours, hovercraft approx. 35 mins. Arrive Paris, Gare du Nord late afternoon or early evening and transfer by coach to your hotel. Return similar timings arriving London afternoon or evening.

ITINERARY: Paris Coach Express

Depart London (King's Cross Coach Terminal) at 9.30a.m. Friday for Dover. Ship crossing approx. 1½ hours. Arrive Paris hotel approx. 10p.m. Three nights hotel. Saturday morning tour of Paris and afternoon visit to Versailles also included. Return London late Monday, approx. 10p.m.

Assignment 26: A new image for the salon

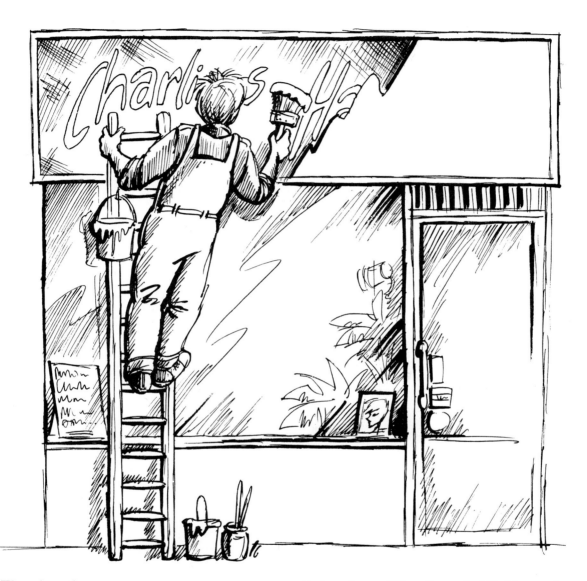

The situation

You have just started work in a hair and beauty salon recently taken over by a bright and imaginative young couple anxious to change their establishment from a rather dull and staid one to a salon catering especially for the 16 to 25 age group of both sexes. Your employers have asked you to help them give their salon a 'New Image'. *NB* Money is, on this occasion, no object!

Task 1

Make a list of all the things you would have to consider, e.g. layout of furniture, when making the transformation.

Task 2

Design an advertisement to go in the local newspaper or magazine.

Task 3

Design a price list for display in the salon.

Task 4

Design an appointments card.

Task 5

Produce a one-minute advertising script for your local radio station.

Assignment 27: The faulty scissors

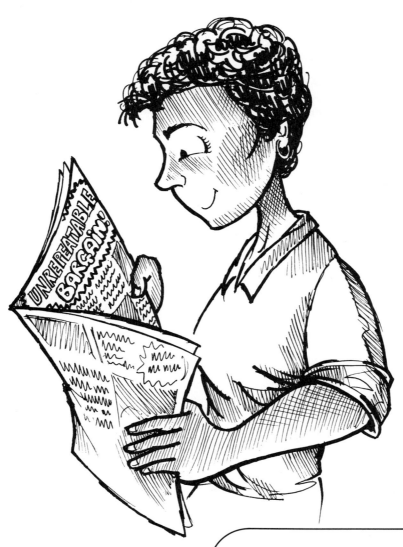

The situation

You have just been given a job as a junior trainee in a local hairdressing salon. One morning during your 'break' you are looking through a hairdressing magazine when you see the following advertisement:

Task 1

This appears to be a very good offer, and you decide to order a set of these scissors. Write an appropriate letter to 'Hairdressers' Snips Ltd.'.

Task 1

The scissors arrive and at first you are very pleased with them. After one week, however, you discover a bad fault in one of the pairs and decide to return them and ask for your money back. Write a letter of complaint to 'Hairdressers' Snips Ltd.'.

Task 3

Write back an appropriate letter of apology from the Sales Manager of 'Hairdressers' Snips Ltd.', who is genuinely keen to please his customers and to build up a high reputation for his newly established company.

Assignment 28: The mobile hairdresser

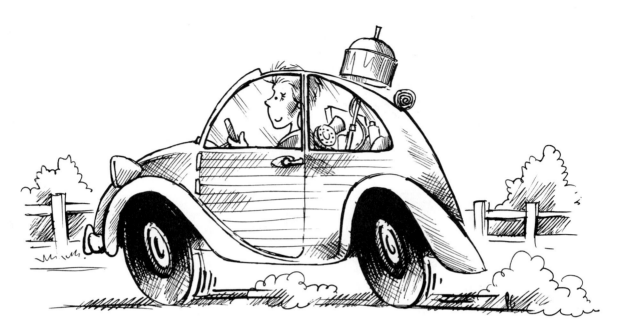

The situation

Many hairdressers start their careers by working as mobile hairdressers. Imagine that you are one, and have six clients to deal with on one particular day.

1 Sophie, who is 3 years old and who simply needs a basic trim.
2 Rick, the punk, who is at home recovering from an operation. He wants his hair shaved back into a Mohican. His girl friend is coming to visit him at 3 o'clock and he wants to give her a surprise.
3 Hilary, who works in a day nursery. She wants a cut and blow dry and is going out to a disco in the evening.
4 Old Mrs Mason, who needs a shampoo and set, and
5 Her unemployed grandson, Kevin, who wants a burgundy rinse.
6 Sharon, who wants her hair highlighted on her half day.

Task 1

Look at the street map and work out your programme for the day.
(a) Make a timetable for the day
(b) Explain the route you would take to visit each client.

Task 2

You ask your clients if you can leave them your card and price list to show their friends (a good way of building up a business). Design your own card and price list.

Task 3

Write a letter to a friend in hospital telling her about your day's work.

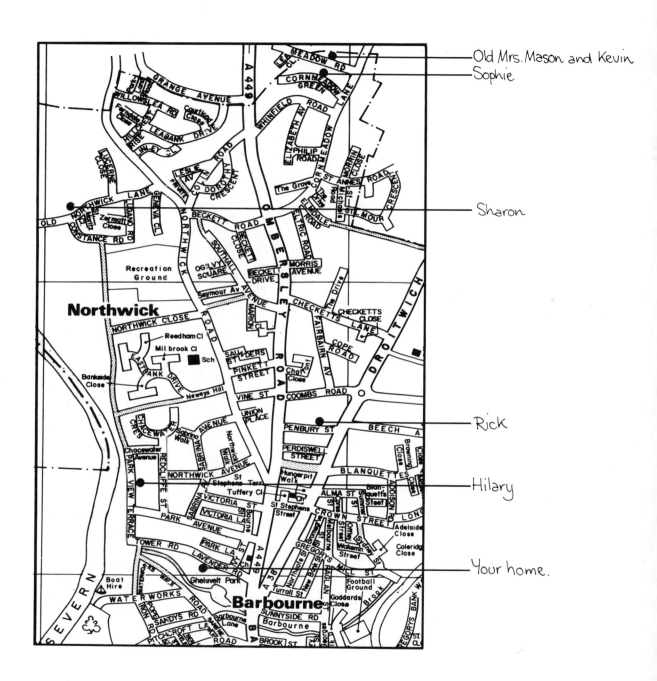

Old Mrs. Mason and Kevin

Sophie

Sharon

Rick

Hilary

Your home.

Assignment 29: Make-up girls on location

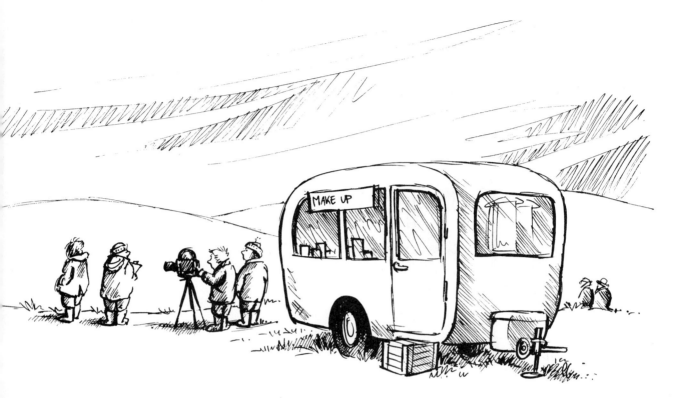

Please read the following passage carefully:

On location

At eight-o-clock on a raw, wintry, North Yorkshire morning the cluster of buildings and fields known to millions of viewers as *Emmerdale Farm* has nothing of the glamour which people often assume to be associated with making television programmes on location. A heavy frost, a stinging north-east wind and the promise of sleet to come, soon remind early arrivals that television is a job, and that creating make-believe often has the icy touch of reality about it.

Already the generator which supplies power to the OB unit is humming away, and a light flickers on in the make-up caravan as the two girls arrive and set out their equipment. Make-up girls insist that their job is not glamorous, despite the popular image to the contrary. They point out that it is always tiring, rarely comfortable, and sometimes downright unpleasant. At 8 am on a February morn, who could argue? Their first task on arriving at the caravan is to plug in the heated

rollers and brushes ready for the first of the artistes to arrive at around 8.30 am. Then they set out their equipment, towels, soaps, shavers, lotions, creams, powders and so on. The caravan is supplied with hot and cold running water, of course, and plenty of lighting, for make-up must be performed under the most searching of lights.

It takes them around half-an-hour on average to make up the female artists; about half that time for the men. Specialised work, however, can take three hours or more, and if blood is needed — they make their own! There are fourteen main characters in the programme and over the years the make-up girls get to know them very well, with all the plusses and minuses which attend familiarity. The girls get to know the idiosyncrasies of each artiste and the requirements of the character he or she plays. Make-up girls are extremely discreet. They have to be, for not only do they see the weaknesses and flaws of the 'stars', but there are even more intimate exchanges of confidences between them than those traditionally made between the housewife and the hairdresser.

They are always expected to be cheerful, well groomed and tireless, and this, paradoxically, they find one of the most tiring aspects of their work. They would not be in the profession if they had a dislike of people, and they usually are to be found smiling, raising morale, and rebuilding confidence with their personality and make-up skills.

Not all *Emmerdale Farm* locations are centred around the site of the farm itself, so when the OB unit moves on they gather their boxes of equipment and follow. At the new location there might be a caravan for them, perhaps the 'snug' of a pub, perhaps a room in a cottage borrowed for the day in which to carry on their work.

Having made up the artistes, their job is not over. They must be in attendance at each scene, tramping across fields and streams with the rest of the team, to check the make-up at the end of each 'take' and to repair and renew any 'damage'. They, too, must be aware of the need to maintain continuity, so they take polaroid pictures of any specialised make-up which must be repeated on another day at another location.

Creative they must be. Yet they must also be practical, resilient and not a little diplomatic. But in their caravan this freezing, February morning their thoughts are directed only at the day ahead. They will be on their feet much of the time, tending to their charges as they follow one another into the little hut. 'Could someone fetch us a coffee, please?'

Note: OB — Outside Broadcast.

From *Television — Behind the Scenes*, Peter Jones (Blandford Press, 1984).

Task 1

Now answer the following questions:
1 Explain the term 'On location'.
2 At what time of day and at what time of the year are these location shots being made?
3 How would the 'make-up girls' describe their work?
4 What do the girls have to do first?
5 How long, on average does it take to make-up the artistes?
6 What do you understand by the term 'specialised work'? Can you give any examples?
7 Why do the make-up girls have to be 'extremely discreet'?
8 What aspect of their work do the make-up girls find the most tiring?
9 Explain the use of the words 'take', 'damage' and 'continuity' in the next to last paragraph.
10 What 4 words summarise the qualities needed for a make-up artist?

Task 2

Write a clear account of how you would set about the make-up design for a television programme of your own choosing. Give reasons for your choice.

Assignment 30: Setting up on your own

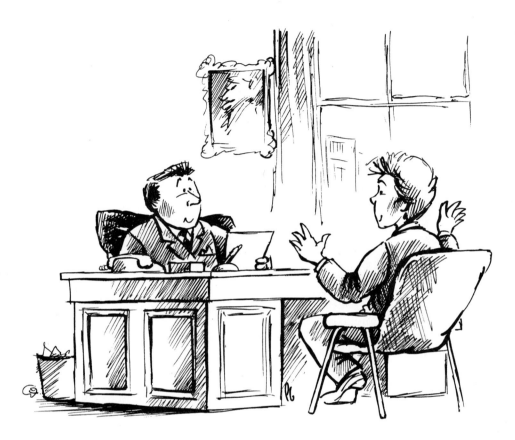

Introduction

All hairdressing and beauty therapy students dream of the day when they are running their own salon. There are 2 ways of achieving this:
1 By buying premises outright and in your own name.
2 By buying the franchise (the right to set up an identical operation to an existing successful one, using the established name of the original one). The buyer also benefits from back-up services such as advertising, financial advice and marketing. The deal usually involves the initial purchase price of the franchise and then paying back a percentage of the takings. Wimpy is probably one of the largest franchises in this country and the chain Command Perfor-

mance hairdressing salons is hoping to expand in the UK, following successful operation in the USA.

If you are thinking of buying a franchise, your main concern (unless you are lucky and money is no problem) will be finding the initial price, but if you are hoping to buy your own premises in your own name there are a number of very important factors to consider.

1 *Location of premises*
This is perhaps the most important factor of all and one which can cause the failure or success of the operation. The location determines what sort of client you are going to attract, although reputation is equally important here.

2 Finance

Apart from the wide range of Government-backed schemes to help small businesses, there are 3 principal ways of raising a loan:

(a) a bank

(b) a Building Society

(c) a Finance Company such as Mercantile Credit.

All 3 need to be looked at closely, and obviously a personal discussion with the manager would be necessary before a large sum of money could be loaned.

3 The Premises

Will you have to spend a large amount of money on alterations? Are there facilities for car parking? Is there room for expansion if necessary? When you consider all these factors you will need the services of:

4 Professional Advisers

(a) Accountant, who will advise you on all aspects of finance.

(b) Solicitor, who will prepare any necessary legal documents or agreements (lease or purchase of premises, franchise, etc.)

(c) Surveyor, who will give advice on suitability of premises and carry out a structural survey.

(c) Architect, who will carry out design work and prepare any necessary drawings and specifications for alterations to the premises.

(e) Insurance broker, who will advise on all aspects of insurance.

Remember — all these people, except the insurance broker, will charge a professional fee for their services.

NB Your regional office of the Department of Trade will give you details of Government schemes to help small businesses.

There is also a whole range of very useful handbooks on the subject which are well worth reading and which would be very helpful to someone 'setting up on their own'.

The situation

You have inherited a small amount of money from a distant relative and decide to add it to your savings and 'set up on your own'. (The sum involved is for you to decide but it will be necessary to borrow a fairly large sum in order to fulfil your dream.)

Task 1

Either by direct approach to an Estate Agent, or by writing, obtain details of possible premises.

Task 2

Prepare a report for your Bank Manager, which you hope will persuade him that you have a potentially successful business in mind, so that he will agree to his bank offering you a loan to fund the project.